"This wonderful, practical resource provides a much needed 'union' between the practices of speech-language pathology and yoga. Whether it's a quick breathing exercise or yoga pose within a therapy session, or a full classroom-based storybook yoga lesson, children are sure to progress in their speech, language, literacy, and pretend play development."

—*Susan Hendler Lederer, PhD, CCC, Professor, Speech-Language Pathologist, yogi, and certified children's yoga instructor*

"This wonderful, comprehensive map of speech and language development in children is a beautifully crafted guide with thoughtful, creative ideas and suggestions for using yoga to facilitate communication skills. An artful blend of science, experience, and wisdom. I will recommend this inspiring book to my SLP students, to parents and caregivers, and to fellow yogis."

—*Kathy Downing, MA, CCC, Speech-Language Pathologist, lecturer, Queens College, City University of New York, prana yoga teacher*

"This is a fantastic guide for parents wondering if yoga is right for their children. The authors explain key aspects of child development, and how to make yoga a fun, valuable experience. As a yogi and a mom who practices with my own kids, I am grateful for this 'go to' resource."

—*Courtney, yoga practitioner and mom of two*

"*Yoga for Speech-Language Development* shatters the notion that yoga should be reserved as a 'quiet time' activity in the early childhood classroom. This is a compelling look at the lyrical, whimsical, and playful components of yogic principals and how they can provide the perfect arena for supporting reciprocal and engaging communication with the young child."

—*Peggy Natale, Program Director, SteppingStone Day School*

of related interest

Building Language Using LEGO® Bricks
A Practical Guide
Dawn Ralph and Jacqui Rochester
Foreword by Gina Gómez De La Cuesta
ISBN 978 1 78592 061 5
eISBN 978 1 78450 317 8

Asanas for Autism and Special Needs
Yoga to Help Children with their Emotions,
Self-Regulation and Body Awareness
Shawnee Thornton Hardy
ISBN 978 1 84905 988 6
eISBN 978 1 78450 059 7

Yoga Therapy for Every Special Child
Meeting Needs in a Natural Setting
Nancy Williams
Illustrated by Leslie White
ISBN 978 1 84819 027 6
eISBN 978 0 85701 027 8

YOGA
for
SPEECH-LANGUAGE
DEVELOPMENT

SUSAN E. LONGTIN AND
JESSICA A. FITZPATRICK

Illustrations by Michelle Mozes

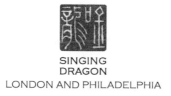

SINGING
DRAGON
LONDON AND PHILADELPHIA

Every effort has been made to trace copyright holders and to obtain their permission for the use of copyright material. The author and the publisher apologize for any omissions and would be grateful if notified of any acknowledgements that should be incorporated in future reprints or editions of this book.

Page 12: The B.K.S. Iyengar quotation has been reproduced with permission from p.76 of *Astadala Yogamala* Volume 1 by B.K.S. Iyengar published by Allied Publishers Private Limited in 2000. Page 24: The Janice Light quotation "Communication is the essence of human life" appears in the title of an article by Janice Light published in 1997 in the journal *Augmentative and Alternative Communication 13* (2) and has been reproduced with permission. Page 26: Figure 2.1 has been reproduced with permission from Figure 1 on p.14 in the 2001 Monograph for the Society for Research on Children Development called *The Intentionality Model and Language Acquisition* by Lois Bloom and Erin Tinker, published by Wiley. Page 68: Permission for the Dan Brulé quotation has been kindly granted by Dan Brulé (www.breathmastery.com, author of *Just Breathe: Mastering Breathwork for Success in Life, Love, Business, and Beyond*). Page 106: The Jean Piaget quotation has been reproduced with permission from *Play, Dreams, and Imitation in Childhood* by Jean Piaget published in 1962 by W.W. Norton.

First published in 2017
by Singing Dragon
an imprint of Jessica Kingsley Publishers
73 Collier Street
London N1 9BE, UK
and
400 Market Street, Suite 400
Philadelphia, PA 19106, USA

www.singingdragon.com

Copyright © Susan E. Longtin and Jessica A. Fitzpatrick 2017
Illustrations copyright © Michelle Mozes 2017
Front cover image source: Michelle Mozes

Library of Congress Cataloging in Publication Data
Title: Yoga for speech-language development / Susan E. Longtin and Jessica A. Fitzpatrick ; illustrations by Michelle Mozes.
Description: London ; Philadelphia : Jessica Kingsley Publishers, 2017. | Includes bibliographical references and index.
Identifiers: LCCN 2016042441 | ISBN 9781848192584 (alk. paper)
Subjects: | MESH: Speech Therapy--methods | Yoga | Language Development | Child
Classification: LCC RC423 | NLM WL 340.3 | DDC 616.85/5062--dc23 LC record available at https://lccn.loc.gov/2016042441

British Library Cataloguing in Publication Data
A CIP catalogue record for this book is available from the British Library

ISBN 978 1 84819 258 4
eISBN 978 0 85701 205 0

Printed and bound in Great Britain

Acknowledgements

We would like to acknowledge our BambooMoves yoga community in Forest Hills, New York, especially Suzanne Scholten, Ora Sukov, Jennifer Fink, and Jennifer Pinna for sharing their knowledge, skills, and resources with us. We also wish to acknowledge Alyssa Dreifus and Zarema Ibadullayeva from Brooklyn College/City University of New York for their assistance in compiling the yoga resources that appear in the Appendix of this book.

Contents

PART III: APPENDICES OF YOGA RESOURCES

Disclaimer

Throughout this book we made the arbitrary decision to use the traditionally feminine pronouns "she," "her," and "hers" to designate a variety of adults that could be male or female—parents, teachers, and therapists. Consequently, we decided to use the traditionally male pronouns "he," "him," and "his" to designate infants and children. We chose these pronoun designations to avoid having to use the awkward forms "he/she," "him/her," and "his/hers" to refer to children in this book.

Whether male or female, we firmly believe that all children are unique with their own profiles and develop at their own pace. Children also vary in strength, flexibility, and balance. This principle of individual variation applies to children who are typically developing as well as those with developmental challenges. Children in this latter group may also present with deep, focused interests, sensory profiles, motor skills, and attentional capacities that impact their participation in a yoga practice. The adult who guides children will need to take these individual differences into account and adapt the yoga poses and breathing exercises to meet their unique needs. The adult who engages in yoga with children with developmental challenges needs to be knowledgeable of the children's capacities and modify the practice accordingly.

This book contains illustrations of children and parent-child dyads engaged in yoga poses. These illustrations were designed to enhance the text and provide idealized representations of the poses. They do not depict any particular individual's expression of the pose. In fact, some children (or adults) may not be able to achieve the alignment demonstrated in the illustrations, which are intended to assist the adult in visualizing the form of a yoga pose, rather than its absolute representation.

This book contains an Appendix of books, card decks, CDs, DVDs, games, and web-based resources. These resources could be incorporated into individual or group children's yoga sessions as the adult sees fit. The resource list, while extensive, is not exhaustive. Consequently, some noteworthy children's yoga resources may have been unintentionally omitted from the list. In addition, the authors of this book do not endorse these resources nor have they obtained any compensation to promote them. Rather, they are simply provided to assist the adult who wishes to explore them, and then decide those that they might use.

Throughout this book, the authors highlight logical connections between yoga and the development of speech, language, and communication, but currently no direct research evidence supports the use of yoga to enhance speech-language development in children. The authors hope that their demonstration of and commitment to these connections will encourage a first genera-tion of research-oriented yoga practitioners and clinicians to gather preliminary data on these relations.

PART I

INTRODUCTION

Chapter 1

YOGA AND ITS RELATION TO SPEECH-LANGUAGE DEVELOPMENT

Yoga, an ancient but perfect science, deals with the evolution of humanity. This evolution includes all aspects of one's being, from bodily health to self-realization. Yoga means union—the union of body with consciousness and consciousness with the soul. Yoga cultivates the ways of maintaining a balanced attitude in day-to-day life and endows skill in the performance of one's actions.

B.K.S. Iyengar

Introduction to yoga

The word yoga comes from the Sanskrit word "*yuj*" meaning to yoke or bind. Yoga is the union of the body, mind, and spirit. Since yoga was initially passed down from teacher to student by oral tradition, the exact origin of yoga in ancient India is unknown. Approximately 2000 years ago (Goldberg 2013), the great sage Patanjali systematized the philosophy and practice of yoga. *The Yoga Sutras of Patanjali* (Satchidananda 2011) contain insights for achieving this union of the mind, body, and spirit. This work describes the eight limbs or steps of yoga, which provide guidelines for living a full, purposeful, content life. Three of these practices—

the poses, breathing exercises, and meditation—comprise the main parts of yoga, which are represented in Figure 1.1.

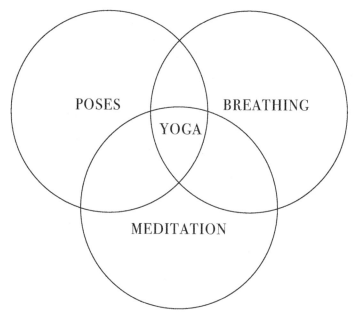

Figure 1.1 Three main parts of yoga: poses, breathing, and meditation

Yoga poses

The first component of yoga, the physical poses, improves overall strength, flexibility, and balance. Yoga poses can be categorized as standing, balancing, twisting, hip opening, bending, and inverting. Figure 1.2 illustrates these six categories of poses.

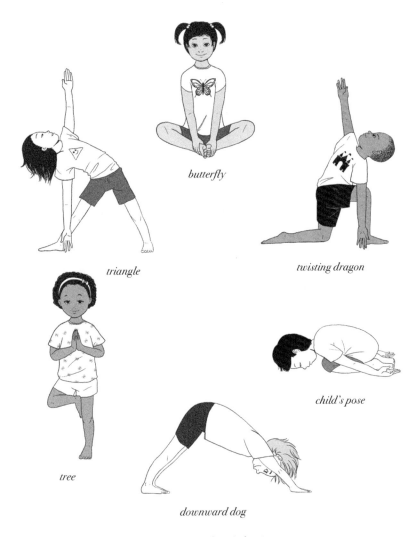

butterfly

triangle

twisting dragon

child's pose

tree

downward dog

Figure 1.2 Six categories of yoga poses: standing, balancing, twisting, hip opening, bending, and inverting

Standing poses, such as triangle pose, teach proper alignment of the body and feet, improving posture. Standing poses also ground and connect practitioners to the earth. Balancing poses, such as tree pose, tone muscles, elongate the spine, and improve body posture too. These poses require significant concentration, which help keep the mind focused in the present moment. Twisting poses, such as twisting dragon, release tension and lengthen the spine, increase shoulder and hip mobility, and stretch the back muscles. As the trunk of the body turns, twists activate kidney and abdominal organs to improve digestion and remove sluggishness in all the bodily systems. Hip opening poses, such as butterfly, promote proper alignment of the sacrum and pelvis so that practitioners can sit, walk, and move with greater comfort and ease. Hip opening poses alleviate stress, calm the nervous system, and combat fatigue. Hip openers are also important for practicing safe, deep forward and backward bends, as well as for sitting comfortably for meditation.

Forward bends, such as child's pose, stretch the lower back and hamstrings, release tension in the upper body, and increase spinal flexibility. They also promote a calm, relaxed state. Backward bends, such as camel pose, open the chest and hips, strengthen the arms and shoulders, and increase the flexibility of the spine. Backward bends also stimulate the nervous system and clear the mind of extraneous thoughts. Inverted poses, such as downward facing dog, build strength and endurance in the upper body, as well as stimulate the brain. When the legs are positioned higher than the heart, the flow of blood and other fluids in the body reverses, relieving tension in the legs.

The different categories of yoga poses are not mutually exclusive as some of them can belong to more than one category. For example, "tree" is a standing, balancing, and hip opening pose. The ultimate goal of all the yoga poses is to prepare the body for stillness and meditation.

Yogic breathing

The second component of yoga, the breathing exercises, focuses on control over the breath. Certain breathing exercises calm the body, whereas others energize it. During a yoga practice it is important to synchronize the breath with the poses. For example, backward bending poses occur on inhalation, and forward bending poses occur on exhalation. Coordination of the breath with the yoga poses allows increased blood flow and oxygenation in the body (Williams 2010). A well-oxygenated body, and specifically brain, may positively impact overall learning.

In the west, hatha yoga is the most commonly known form of yoga. The word "*ha*" means sun, and "*tha*" means moon. Hatha yoga seeks to unite these opposite forces and find balance. Hatha yoga is the physical practice of the poses in conjunction with the breath. It involves safely challenging the body in poses while keeping the breath steady to find the balance between effort and ease. Proper alignment of the parts of the body opens the energy channels, especially the main energy channel in the spine. This results in a strong, flexible, balanced body, which leads to a balanced mind.

Yogic meditation

During meditation, the third component of yoga, the focus shifts from the distractions of the external world to the silence of the inner one. Concentration is the beginning of meditation. Concentration on an "object," such as a sound, candle flame, or picture, can provide a single point of focus to begin meditation. Another path to meditation is the practice of "mindfulness," which involves the nonjudgmental observation of thoughts, feelings, bodily sensations, and the surrounding environment from moment to moment (Alkalay 2001). Originally an ancient Buddhist tradition, mindfulness has become a popular contemporary subject of investigation and discussion, especially in the field of psychology. In 1979, researcher and leader in the area of mindfulness, Jon Kabat-Zinn, introduced his Mindfulness-Based Stress Reduction (MBSR) program at the University of Massachusetts Medical School. Since then, numerous studies have documented the physical and mental benefits of MBSR and mindfulness in general. The National Scientific Council of the Developing Child states that excessive stress damages children's developing brain, which leaves them susceptible to learning, behavior, and health issues. Fortunately, evidence is building that the mindfulness practice present in yoga is an effective way to promote healthy brain development and function, as well as stress relief (Flynn 2013; Flynn and Ebert 2013). Current research also shows that teaching mindfulness in the classroom reduces aggression and other challenging behaviors while increasing calmness and concentration. Furthermore, scientific research indicates that mindfulness practice increases the density of gray matter in brain areas linked to learning, memory, emotion regulation, and empathy (Greater Good Science Center, University of California, Berkeley n.d.).

In summary, yoga strengthens the connection between the body, mind, and spirit. With a strong, flexible body and balanced mind, the practitioner connects to the inner spirit. Additionally, through a consistent yoga practice involving all three components—poses, breathwork, and meditation—the practitioner creates space for acquiring new ideas.

Yoga and speech-language development

Contemporary interest in and research on yoga has increased in recent years. The fields of medicine, education, physical therapy, occupational therapy, and psychotherapy embraced yoga, which is recognized by the United States National Institutes of Health (NIH) as a complementary, integrative treatment method. The National Center for Complementary and Integrative Health (NCCIH) of the NIH provides a list of selected references on this topic.

The benefits of yoga for adults are documented in the scientific literature (e.g. Broad 2012; Lee 2006; McCall 2007; Yurtkuran *et al.* 2007). Growing evidence suggests that, like adults, children benefit from practicing yoga. The emerging evidence-base for the benefits of yoga with children consists of systematic reviews (e.g. Birdee *et al.* 2009; Galantino, Galbavy, and Quinn 2008; Kaley-Isley *et al.* 2010; Serwacki and Cook-Cottone 2012), randomized controlled trials (e.g. Jensen and Kenny 2004; White 2012), pretest-posttest efficacy studies (e.g. Eggleston 2015; Koenig, Buckley-Reen, and Garg 2012), feasibility studies (e.g. Thygeson *et al.* 2010), descriptive research (e.g. Harper 2010; White 2012), and anecdotal reports (Flynn and Ebert 2013). This literature suggests that yoga benefits children with respect to psycho-physiological outcomes, such as stress reduction (Eggleston 2015; White 2012), as well as increased self-regulation (Ehleringer 2010; Kenny 2002), attention (Ehleringer 2010; Jensen and Kenny 2004), and self-esteem (Eggleston 2015). Research has documented the educational and therapeutic benefits from the fields of education, physical therapy, occupational therapy, medicine, and psychotherapy. Some studies claim that children who received yoga as a rehabilitative adjunct to traditional physical (Galantino *et al.* 2008) and occupational (Koenig *et al.* 2012) therapies benefitted from the practice. However, researchers, including those who have conducted systematic reviews of the evidence, agree that additional research is needed. More rigorous research designs with larger clinical trials are required to support the use of yoga with both typically developing and disordered populations of children.

The practice of yoga in school settings has become increasingly popular over the past decade with an accumulation of the scientific evidence for this trend. When yoga is used in schools, the focus is typically on educating the whole child and includes areas such as improving test anxiety, stress resilience, concentration, well-being, and self-esteem (Butzer *et al.* 2015; Eggleston 2015; Flynn and Ebert 2013). Several manualized, research-based programs for elementary school children have been developed and evaluated in recent years. For example, evaluation of the *Yoga 4 Schools®* program (Hyde 2012) indicated that through their participation in this program, typically developing elementary school students improved their self-esteem, physical health, and academic performance. For another example, evaluation of the *Get Ready to Learn* program, which targeted challenging behaviors in students with autism spectrum disorder (ASD) (Koenig *et al.* 2012), indicated that those students who participated in this yoga program reduced their irritability, social withdrawal, hyperactivity, and noncompliance.

In addition to yoga for the school-age years, programs have been developed for the infant-toddler and preschool populations. *Baby Om* and *ChildLight Yoga* are two examples of such programs. Children at these younger ages are in the peak speech-language learning years. It is our position that yoga practices for these age groups can support speech-language development.

As speech-language pathologists, we have noted that yogic principles and practices have been used to treat the speech disorder of stuttering (Balakrishnan 2009; Boyle 2011; Kauffman *et al.* 2010). It is also common practice in voice therapy to incorporate breath control (Gilman 2014) and vocal relaxation techniques, which are used in yoga. However, beyond stuttering and voice disorders, applications of yoga in the field of speech-language pathology have been limited. We acknowledge that the research to support the evidence-base for the direct use of yoga to enhance speech-language development has not been conducted. However, we firmly believe that the connections between certain yoga practices and speech-language and play development are sufficiently compelling.

This book addresses the logical relations between yoga and child speech-language development in different domains and at various stages. We propose that yoga can enhance speech, language, cognition, and play skills throughout the developmental periods. Yoga can enhance the prelinguistic communication skills of eye gaze, joint attention, and turn-taking in infants and toddlers. These skills, which reflect the children's engagement with their caretakers, are the foundation for future communicative interactions. For example, turn-taking with vocalizations and toys during the first two years of life is the foundation for conversational turn-taking at later stages of development. The parent-child yoga classes for infants and toddlers provide many opportunities for engagement and prelinguistic communication.

The prelinguistic stage is followed by the emergence of early speech and language. Speech refers to the sounds emitted through the oral and nasal cavities and takes shape in the form of words (Hamaguchi 2010). Yoga, with its emphasis on the coordination of breath with movement, can enhance breath support for speech. Breath support involves stabilizing the body for proper airflow. Practicing the yoga poses helps stabilize the body. With the body strong in proper alignment, speech, which occurs on exhaled air, becomes more efficient.

Yoga can facilitate the motor act of speaking. The brain sends signals to the muscles that control the articulators, namely the tongue, lips, and jaw, to produce clear, connected speech. Two yoga practices, the poses and chanting (sound sequences), require motor planning, or praxis. The poses require motor planning at the level of the body while chanting involves motor planning for speech. Sequencing movements for speech is important for generating meaningful spoken language. Repetition of the poses and chants provides opportunities for children to practice and eventually master these different motor plans.

Yoga can help children build their vocabulary and linguistic concepts. By five years of age children understand at least 10,000 words and use at least 900–2000 words (Shipley and McAfee 2009).

Yoga exposes children to different types of words including nouns, pronouns, verbs, adjectives, adverbs, and prepositions. Many of these words express linguistic concepts, which describe location (e.g. "in front of" and "behind"), quantity (e.g. "less" and "more"), attributes (e.g. "little" and "big"), time (e.g. "before" and "after"), and feelings (e.g. "happy" and "sad"). In terms of comprehension, the practice of yoga allows children the opportunity to follow directions involving these different linguistic concepts.

Yoga can enhance emergent literacy skills in preschool-aged children. Many children's books, especially those that feature animals, present opportunities to practice yoga poses. The emergent literacy skill of phonological awareness involves playing with sounds and words, such as creating rhymes. Chanting provides an opportunity for children to play with different sounds and syllabic structures. Phonological awareness skills are important predictors for learning to read. In addition to supporting emergent literacy, shared book reading provides a context in which to enhance communication between adults and children, through joint attention, as well as facilitate many other aspects of language including following directions, vocabulary and concepts acquisition, and sentence development.

Play is a domain of development that is related to language. This connection is seen as the child moves from the late toddler stage into the preschool years. Piaget (1962) proposed that play and language in children are both examples of the symbolic function, which involves using one object to stand for another. Through yoga poses, children use their physical bodies in playful ways to represent different animals, such as a lion, and objects, such as a table. Children learn language through play. Play is so important for young children's development that it is considered the *work* of childhood!

Executive functions have been the area most frequently researched in the clinical/educational literature on the benefits of yoga for children. While the topic of executive functions will not be directly addressed in this book, these skills are related to language. Attention, memory, planning, organization, and regulation are examples of executive functions. Children, particularly in school settings, are required to sit still and attend for long periods of time. However, children are rarely taught *how* to sit quietly and listen. Yoga teaches children how to control their bodies and breathe so that they can pay attention to learning tasks (Goldberg 2013). The practice of yoga provides children with opportunities to attend to other people, including their teachers, caregivers, and peers. It requires remembering and executing sequences of movements for the poses, breathing exercises, and chants. Meditation and mindfulness practices help children maintain a calm, organized, and regulated state (Flook *et al.* 2010). Executive functions are critical for learning to think, act, and solve problems in everyday life.

Yoga can also be used to enhance speech-language development in children diagnosed with different neurodevelopmental disabilities including language disorders, speech sound disorders, intellectual disabilities, ASD, and attention deficit/hyperactivity disorders (AD/HD). Children with these conditions can feel frustrated when they are unable to express themselves in an effective, appropriate manner. Yoga provides a relaxed, playful environment that stimulates communication and social exchanges (Flynn and Ebert 2013; Goldberg 2013; Williams 2010). Yoga instruction for children involves modeling and multisensory cueing, including verbal, visual, and tactile-kinesthetic cues, to carry out the poses, breathing exercises, and meditation practices. In both children with and without neurodevelopmental disabilities, yoga can enhance breath support and motor planning for speech, vocabulary and concept development, emergent literacy skills, and symbolic play. These aspects of development will be explored in greater detail in the subsequent chapters.

Summary

Yoga is an ancient tradition that consists of the three practices of poses, breathing exercises, and meditation. The six non-mutually exclusive categories of yoga poses include standing, balancing, twisting, hip opening, bending, and inverting. Yogic breath focuses on control and coordination of the breath cycle with movement and a type of speech called chants. Meditation shifts the practitioner from the external to the internal world begun by concentrating on a single point of focus. The popular practice of "mindfulness," the here-and-now nonjudgmental observation of one's thoughts, feelings, and sensations, is a pathway to meditation that promotes healthy brain development and stress relief according to current research. The use of yoga with adults is a well-established complementary and alternative approach to health and well-being. Yoga for children has increased exponentially over the past decade and has been embraced by educators and clinicians in various fields such as psychology as well as physical and occupational therapies. In this book, the focus is on a relatively unexplored area, the use of yoga to support different aspects of children's speech-language development and the related area of play.

Chapter 2

A DEVELOPMENTAL PERSPECTIVE ON LANGUAGE ACQUISITION

Communication is the essence of human life.

Janice Light

Introduction to language development

The acquisition of language is perhaps the most remarkable milestone in early childhood development. Parents and other caregivers often wait expectantly for their child's first word. During the first year of life, before the seemingly miraculous appearance of first words, infants develop several notable capacities that precede and are necessary for language to emerge.

Before proceeding with the models and stages of language acquisition, it must be noted that all aspects of children's development are influenced by their culture (Shonkoff and Phillips 2000), which consists of rules for what is considered appropriate behavior. Culture is learned and used by individuals, including children and their caregivers, as a consequence of belonging to a particular community or group (Saville-Troike 2003). Culture includes values and beliefs that influence all aspects of development—feeding, sleep patterns, parental responsiveness to crying, and role expectations of different family members including parents and grandparents. Speech, language, and communication for all children develop within this cultural context. Children learn language in the context of interacting with others in their communities, which accounts for the variations that occur in children from diverse cultural-linguistic backgrounds. Culture influences many aspects of language development including caregiver-child interaction, which effects the social organization of these exchanges, the value of talk, and beliefs about intentionality and language teaching (Johnston and Wong 2002; Taylor 1999; van Kleeck 1994). Of note, most of the literature on child language development comes from samples of middle-class children of European descent and the descriptions provided here are based primarily on those samples.

Developmental models

When infants are born into this world, they do not have the intention to share meanings through gestures or words. Despite the infants' lack of intentionality, parents or other caretakers are often willing and eager to interpret their infant's movements and sounds as meaningful and communicative. Bloom and Tinker (2001) described an integrative model that captures the unfolding of the infants' intentional states over the first year of life before the emergence of language at the beginning of the second year. Their model, aptly called *the Intentionality Model*, is relevant to the understanding of yogic practices for infants' and toddlers' speech-language development. The model describes how the infants develop the ability to interpret (or understand) and express (through affect, play, and speech) their intentional states, which include beliefs, desires, and feelings about people, objects, and events. The infants' acts of interpreting (or understanding) lay the groundwork for their comprehension and communication through language. Figure 2.1 displays a diagram illustrating the components of the Intentionality Model and the interactions among them.

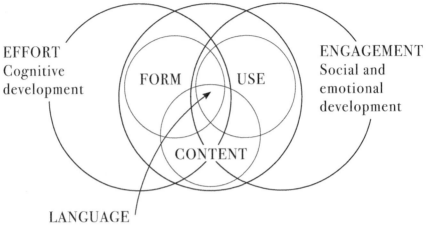

Figure 2.1 The Intentionality Model

From "The intentionality model and language acquisition" by Bloom, L. and Tinker, E. (2001) *Monographs of the Society for Research in Child Development 66*, 4, Serial No. 267, p.14. Copyright 2001 by Blackwell Publishers, a division of John Wiley and Sons, Inc. Reprinted with permission.

The Intentionality Model contains two components, *engagement* and *effort*. Engagement refers to the affective, social-connectedness that infants experience in mutual, reciprocal interactions with others. Infant behaviors such as eye gaze, joint attention, and turn-taking are indications of their engagement with others and provide the foundation of future communicative interactions. Infant-toddler yoga classes offer many opportunities to foster adult-child engagement, which will be discussed in Chapter 4. The second component of the model, effort, refers to the work it takes to learn language. This includes the infants' cognitive resources such as memory as well as the processes of attention, perception, association, and integration. Infant-toddler yoga classes provide many opportunities for the young child to use his cognitive resources and processes as he attends to his caretaker, perceives the events at hand, integrates sights and sounds, and formulates memories of the experience.

Bloom and Lahey (1978) proposed a model of language development that includes three components: form (phonology, morphology, syntax), content (semantics), and use (pragmatics). Language is viewed as the convergence of these three elements. They defined language as a socially shared code or conventional system that represents ideas through the use of arbitrary symbols for communication. This integrative model revolutionized the thinking of speech-language pathologists (SLPs) by providing a "map" of language development, which traced the child's expression of ideas from single words through complex sentences (Gerber and Wankoff 2014). This communication-language orientation (Lahey 1988), based on longitudinal data from typically developing children, provides a developmental-descriptive framework to assist SLPs in determining what children with challenges in learning language should acquire next based on developmental phases. The components of linguistic form, content, and use develop within the broader domains of engagement and effort, components of the Intentionality Model (Figure 2.1), providing a mechanism for continuity between the two models and across developmental stages. In addition, both models view the child's growth across domains as synergistic, with developments occurring simultaneously in multiple domains, such as language content (semantics) and language use (pragmatics). An example of this synergistic, integrative nature of early language is a child who says the word "up" (an example of linguistic form) to code the semantic notion of an action involving a change of place (an example of language content) to request that the adult pick him up (an example of language use). Yoga practices for children, with their emphasis on nurturing the whole child, reflect this synergistic, integrative view of development.

Stages of language development

In this section we describe the stages of language acquisition from a developmental perspective, which espouses that all aspects of the child's development—cognitive, neurobiological, social-emotional, and affective—contribute to the language acquisition process. According to this view, development is both integrative and synergistic across these domains. Gerber and Prizant (2000) provide an overview of seven stages of language development that is consistent with the models described above. Table 2.1 lists a description of each stage. These stages can be used to describe the language development of typically developing children as well as those with challenges in learning to communicate, talk, and understand. Of course, the stages do not begin and end at discrete points, but rather are continuous over time. In addition, children vary in their rate of development so that the amount of time needed to pass from one stage to another differs depending on several factors, such as the child's constitution, temperament, learning capacities, and environment.

Table 2.1 Stages, ages, and characteristics of communication-language development in typically developing children

Stage	Age	Communication-language characteristics
Preintentional	Birth to 8 months	Infants gaze, smile, laugh, touch, grasp, and vocalize to express their feelings and interest in the world; adults interpret their behaviors as communicative.
Prelinguistic Intentional	8–12 months	Infants engage in purposeful, intentional two-way communication through gestures, gaze, and vocalizations.
One-Word Utterances	12–18 months	Toddlers acquire approximately 50 different words, which they use to express basic meanings and communicate with others.

Two-Word Utterances	18–24 months	Toddlers combine words with word-order rules to express basic meanings and communicate with others.
Early Syntactic-Semantic Complexity	2–3½ years	Children produce three-word utterances and early grammatical morphemes to express a greater variety of meanings and communicative functions.
Later Syntactic-Semantic Complexity	3½–7 years	Children produce multiverb utterances and grammatically complex sentences, express more cognitively sophisticated meanings, engage in longer conversations, and tell stories.
Communicative Competence	7–12 years	Children have well-developed syntactic, semantic, and pragmatic skills. Their conversational skills are more advanced, and they vary their language with the communicative context. They understand and produce nonliteral language.

(adapted from Gerber and Prizant 2000)

Individual differences in rate aside, the first stage, the Pre-intentional, begins at birth and lasts until about eight months. The infants' gaze, smiles, laughter, cries, and other vocalizations characterize this prelinguistic stage. Infants express interest in the world of people and objects around them by touching and grasping for objects and by attending to people as social partners. This stage lays the groundwork for the development of comprehension or the understanding of language. Although infants do not have the ability to communicate intentionally during this time period, this stage is noteworthy for adults' frequent responses to infants' behaviors as if they were intentional. For example, a child might gaze and smile at the adult, who attributes the child with having expressed an intention such as being content. The infant might indeed have a feeling of contentedness, but does not intend to express this feeling to the adult for the purpose of communication.

In the next stage of language development, the Prelinguistic Intentional stage, which lasts from about 8 to 12 months, infants acquire the ability to engage in purposeful intentional two-way communication through a variety of nonlinguistic means including gestures, gaze, and vocalizations. For example, the infant might reach or point to a desired object such as a toy on a shelf to request that an adult obtain it. Similarly, a child at this stage could point to a pet dog in order to show it to an adult, a form of early communication called "joint attention." Joint attention is the simultaneous engagement of two (or more) individuals on a single, shared object of focus (Pence Turnbull and Justice 2017). The emergence of joint attention in infants is a hallmark of their development of intentionality. During this first year, infants and their caregivers engage in many everyday routine activities such as mealtime and getting dressed. These everyday routines, called "formats" (Bruner 1983), allow babies to interact with adults in predictable ways. During routines, which are often playful and game-like, infants hear many linguistic form/content/use interactions, which provide opportunities for babies to exercise their receptive language skills.

During this period infants begin to understand words for objects and actions, but only in context. In fact, babies may give the appearance of understanding more than they actually do because of their reliance on comprehension strategies (Weiss 2014) such as looking at the object the adult looks at (Miller and Paul 1995). Young children learn to comprehend language in context, relying on the gestures, objects, and people present. They also rely on what is said in these situations. Consequently, parents and speech-language pathologists often disagree about young children's comprehension (Weiss 2014). Infant-toddler yoga classes have repetitive, routinized scripts and activities that could facilitate language comprehension. For example, during the song, "If You're Happy and You Know It," the caregiver claps the baby's feet or hands together as the relevant word is sung.

At around the time of their first birthday, infants make the transition to language usually producing their first meaningful word. Typically developing one-year-olds might understand about 80 different words whereas they produce only about ten (Pence Turnbull and Justice 2017). The so-called One-Word Stage, which lasts from about 12 to 18 months, is characterized by a slow start and later increased rate of word acquisition. During this time period, many toddlers acquire approximately 50 different words in their expressive vocabularies that can be categorized in different ways. At this stage typically developing children understand many more words than they produce. A comprehension strategy they might use at this stage is to look at the object mentioned by the adult (Miller and Paul 1995).

A traditional description of the words children learn to say and understand classifies them according to various word types such as nouns, verbs, and adjectives. Using this taxonomy, first words include nouns such as "car," verbs such as "go," and adjectives such as "hot." In a broader descriptive system, nouns, main verbs, and adjectives are considered "content" words because used alone they can convey meaning. These content words contrast with "function" words which include copula and auxiliary verbs such as "is" and "are," prepositions such as "in," and conjunctions such as "and." These words that have a primarily grammatical function rarely appear at the earliest stages of language development. Bloom and Lahey (1978) classified early words with another broad system. They divided first words into two categories, namely substantive words, which are primarily nouns, and relational words, which include verbs and adjectives among other word forms. According to this system, young children combine substantive words with relational words once they begin to put together words in the next stage of language development. For example, the substantive word "cookie" can be combined with the relational word "more" to produce the two-word utterance "more cookie."

Another aspect of first words is the meanings or semantic notions that they express. Bloom and Lahey (1978) identified nine broad semantic notions or content categories that were observed during the one-word period of language development. These content categories included the meanings of existence (e.g. "juice"), nonexistence/disappearance (e.g. "gone"), recurrence (e.g. "more"), rejection (e.g. "no"), denial (e.g. "no"), attribution (e.g. "yummy"), possession (e.g. "mine"), action (e.g. "drink"), and locative action (e.g. "out"). As children develop language through the preschool years, they learn to express additional, more cognitively complex semantic notions such as causality. Bloom and Lahey (1978) identified a total of 21 different content categories in children's early language.

Furthermore, as noted in the discussion of the Intentionality Model (Bloom and Tinker 2001), children's language is characterized by the expression of communicative intentions or pragmatic functions. At the One-Word Stage, the toddler uses words to express meaning and intentions. Pragmatic functions at this stage are expressed through words in addition to gestures and nonlinguistic vocalizations. Halliday's (1975) taxonomy of early communicative functions included the instrumental, regulatory, interactional, and personal functions, which could be expressed with a primitive type of language called "protolanguage." This description suggests the continuity between prelinguistic and early linguistic communicative forms and functions. Dore's (1975) primitive speech acts taxonomy, which was developed around the same time, includes functions such as labeling, answering, requesting, calling, greeting, and protesting. Yoga classes for children provide many opportunities for the learning of the three components of linguistic form, content, and use, which will be addressed in the other chapters of this book.

In addition to individual differences in the rate of early language development, variation has also been described in early word forms and functions. Characterizations of these early differences have included Referential and Expressive Styles (Nelson 1973). For example, referential children might tend to use language to label objects in their environment and acquire more noun forms to do so. Expressive children might tend to use language for more personal-social uses and acquire more words for greetings such as "hi" and "bye." The topic of individual differences in early language development is beyond the scope of this chapter, but the interested reader is referred to Goldfield, Snow, and Willenberg (2017) for further information.

By the end of the One-Word Stage, children often combine words to form their first multiword utterances. At this stage, children use language to express different meanings and content categories making a smooth transition into the Two-Word Stage (Gerber and Prizant 2000), which lasts from about 18 to 24 months. During this period, the infant-toddler combines words and shares experiences symbolically. For example, the child could say "drink juice" while pretending to give a doll real or imaginary juice. Of note, the vast majority of the child's word combinations are characterized by correct word order (as in the foregoing example) marking the onset of semantic-syntactic rules in which the child uses word order to express many of the same meanings observed at the One-Word Stage. For example, the child can now say "my juice" instead of being limited to single words such as "mine" or "juice." A marked explosion in both receptive and expressive vocabulary development usually occurs during this time period. In addition, children understand word combinations, simple directions, and wh-questions involving the words "who," "what," and "where"; they comprehend between 150 and

500 words (Miller and Paul 1995). In terms of the use of language, many of the same communicative intentions are expressed at this stage with the emergence of two new functions—the imaginative function to accompany early symbolic play and the informative function in which the child talks about absent objects (Halliday 1975). Dore's (1975) primitive speech act system continues to provide another useful taxonomy for describing children's early communicative intentions at this stage.

Following the Two-Word Stage, children enter the Early Syntactic-Semantic Complexity Stage, which lasts from about two to three-and-a-half years (Gerber and Prizant 2000). Understanding and producing three-word utterances such as "drink more juice" characterize this stage. In these utterances, semantic notions such as action and recurrence are coordinated within the same phrase. Children begin to produce multiverb combinations such as "wanna drink juice." They also begin to use grammatical morphemes such as the present progressive verb inflection to code ongoing action, the plural marker to code quantity, and the words "in" and "on" to code location. At this point in semantic development, young children can talk about many ideas and notions. In terms of the pragmatic use of language, children demonstrate a broad range of communicative functions with the majority of their utterances related to the "here and now." During this stage of development, children might produce utterances such as "I'm putting my blocks in the box" and "That goes here." They use many linguistic verb and noun markers, such as the contractible auxiliary, present progressive verb tense, plural "-s," and third person singular verb marker as in the foregoing examples. At this point, children are capable of producing grammatically complete simple sentences and understand sentences based on morpho-syntactic rules. Children also comprehend a greater variety of question types including "why" and "how many" (Gerber and Prizant 2000; Miller and Paul 1995).

The next stage of language development, called Later Syntactic-Semantic Complexity, occurs between the ages of three-and-a-half to seven years (Gerber and Prizant 2000). During this stage, the children produce multiverb utterances such as "I have to go now" and grammatically complex sentences such as "I have to go now because it's late." At this stage children use this relatively advanced language to talk about more cognitively sophisticated notions as well as events that are removed in time and place. In addition, they understand questions with the terms "how" and "when" and follow multistep directions. They comprehend more locative concepts such as "behind" and "in front of" and the temporal terms "before" and "after" (Gerber and Prizant 2000). By the end of the early childhood years, children understand between 3000 and 8000 words (Miller and Paul 1995).

Children at this stage also produce and understand more varied kinds of discourse including narratives. Children's first stories emerge in a conversational context in interaction with another person during the preschool years forming a type of social monologue. Eventually, by school age, these stories develop into what we typically think of as narratives with a clear beginning, middle, and end. Children's earliest narratives are based on their personal, scripted knowledge derived from previously experienced events such as a doctor's visit or birthday party. Children's later narratives eventually have a defined structure called "story grammar" (Stein and Glenn 1979) with one or more characters and a plot that relates past, present, and future events. The structure of children's narratives varies with their cultural-linguistic background and the stories of children from diverse backgrounds might not adhere to this pattern. Melzi and Schick (2017) provide a discussion on cultural variation in narrative development.

Children achieve the final stage of language development, referred to as Communicative Competence, from 7 to 12 years

(Gerber and Prizant 2000). At this stage children's syntactic, semantic, and pragmatic abilities are well developed. Children have the sophistication to use language in subtle, nuanced ways and to vary their language as a function of the situation at hand. Simply put, they know what to say to whom, when, where, and why. At this stage, children can both understand and produce nonliteral forms of language such as idioms, jokes, and sarcasm. In these forms, the literal meaning does not match the speaker's intended meaning. For example, the idiom "My father hit the roof" means the speaker's father got angry, rather than climbed up to the roof and banged on it. For further information about nonliteral language development in children, the reader is referred to Milosky (1994) and Nippold (2007).

Phonological awareness and emergent literacy

Phonological awareness, an aspect of the development of linguistic form, refers to the ability to focus on the sounds that comprise words and syllables. Phonological awareness is a metalinguistic ability in which the child views the sounds of language as objects of focus. Although predominantly a school-age acquisition, preschoolers manifest some early metalinguistic skills including awareness of rhyme and alliteration. They can identify, blend, and segment sounds in larger units such as syllables and words. These phonological awareness skills are relevant to emergent literacy (Pence Turnbull and Justice 2017), the earliest period that forms the foundation for later reading and writing. This emerging process, which spans the infant, toddler, and preschool years, eventually culminates in the ability to read and write, but, unlike spoken language, requires direct instruction usually from a teacher once children enter school. Emergent literacy, also called the roots of literacy, includes behaviors and skills associated with later successful reading. In addition to phonological awareness, some emergent literacy skills evident before three years (Schickendanz and Collins 2013) include recognizing specific books by cover, pretending to read, turning pages, and listening to stories. Emergent literacy skills evident between the ages of three and four years include knowing that alphabet letters have names, knowing that the information in letters differs from that of pictures, noticing rhyme and alliteration, showing increased interest in books, and connecting stories to life experiences. Yoga classes for children contain enjoyable, playful ways to teach emergent literacy skills to children. Chanting and singing provide opportunities for practicing phonological awareness skills. In addition, yoga poses can be embedded in stories providing a context for the development of other emergent literacy skills, which will be the focus of Chapter 9.

Summary

Language is a complex multidimensional system comprised of the components of form, content, and use. These domains develop in a cultural context in synchrony with one another and with other aspects of development. Language develops after the prelinguistic period of caregiver-child social-emotional engagement and requires the child's cognitive resources, which allow him to attend, perceive, and integrate incoming information from the world. The components of language develop in an integrative, synergistic manner in a stage-like progression through the early childhood years. Language continues to develop during the later school years and adolescence, but these developments are beyond the scope of this book. The reader who wishes to pursue this topic of later language learning is referred to Nippold (2007).

Chapter 3

YOGA FOR DIFFERENT STAGES OF SPEECH-LANGUAGE DEVELOPMENT

Teach what is inside you—not as it applies to you, to yourself, but as it applies to the other.

T. Krishnamacharya

Introduction to yoga for children

A survey conducted by the National Center for Health Statistics revealed a statistically significant increase in the use of yoga from 2.3 percent in 2007 to 3.1 percent in 2012 in children ages 4 to 17 years in the United States (Black *et al.* 2015). Results of a recent survey conducted by *Yoga Journal* and *Yoga Alliance* (2016) indicated that in the United States 36.7 million people reported that they practice yoga, up from the 20.4 million in 2012. The survey also indicated that 37 percent of these practitioners have children under the age of 18 who also practice yoga. The research suggests that yoga's growing popularity is influenced in part by the rise in the number of yoga studios and instructors throughout the country allowing greater accessibility to a larger number of children.

The introduction of yoga to children in their early years leads them on a path of health and well-being. In addition to building strength, balance, and flexibility, the practice of yoga for children presents numerous other physical, cognitive, and emotional benefits. It increases children's awareness of the different parts of their bodies and the various directions in which they move in space. Yoga also increases awareness of breathing, allowing maximum oxygenation and improving overall functioning of bodily systems. Yoga provides opportunities for motor planning, which are necessary for successful execution of sequences of actions. For example, boat pose requires three sequential movements: balancing on the tailbone, elevating the legs, and bringing the arms alongside the body. The practice of yoga improves self-regulation, which is defined as the ability to gain control over bodily functions, manage powerful emotions, and maintain focus and attention (Shonkoff and Phillips 2000). Yogic breathing, chanting, and meditation are particularly beneficial in teaching children to regulate their systems independently. Self-regulation in children is critical for the development of appropriate communication and social skills (Williams 2010), important predictors of later success in life. Although yoga can be practiced *anywhere*, classes in studios, community centers, parks, schools, and other settings led by certified instructors are recommended to learn the techniques needed to build a consistent yoga practice.

Infant-caregiver classes

New mothers and their children from six weeks to one year of age can practice yoga together. Although commonly designated as "Mommy and Baby Yoga" classes, these sessions welcome fathers and other caregivers. Infant-caregiver classes focus on yoga poses that support the development of the important prelinguistic skills of eye gaze, shared attention, and turn-taking. These behaviors are manifestations of the infants' engagement with their caregivers, a topic introduced in the preceding chapter. At this earliest developmental level, the infants' participation in these classes is relatively passive; the caregivers' roles, in contrast, are active. Infants depend on their caregivers to move their bodies into the yoga poses. These movements strengthen infants' muscles, improve their digestion, and facilitate sleep. Research indicates that sleep is critical for the maturation of infants' brains and the integration of their memory networks (Tarullo, Balsam, and Fifer 2011). Researchers found that 15-month-old infants who napped within four hours of exposure to a language sample remembered the general pattern of the sample 24 hours later. In contrast, infants who did not nap shortly following familiarization with the language sample showed no evidence of remembering the pattern (Hupbach *et al.* 2009). Therefore, the sleep benefits of yoga in infants may facilitate language learning.

Toddler classes

When children are considered strong walkers at about 18 to 24 months to approximately three years of age, they become more active participants in yoga classes. Caregivers typically continue to be present in sessions for this age group. Partner poses between children and caregivers offer opportunities for communicative interactions. Children in this age range begin to follow verbal directions that include various linguistic concepts with the support of demonstrations and gestures, providing a context for the development of language comprehension. Concurrently, these toddlers learn to move their bodies independently as they pretend to become elements of nature, such as butterflies, flowers, and waterfalls, in the various poses, which promotes the emergence of symbolic play. This topic will be explored in greater detail in Chapter 8. Yoga classes for children at this level involve breathing exercises that support their developing speech skills; Chapter 5 addresses this topic. Simple chants and songs enhance motor planning for speech, which will be discussed in Chapter 6.

Yoga classes for children at this age also enrich emergent literacy skills, which will be the focus of Chapter 9.

As children learn through repetition, teachers of toddler yoga classes often establish routines to help children learn new skills. For example, classes may consistently begin with a sun salutation adapted for this age group or end with a farewell song, such as "Namaste." Some specialized toddler yoga classes involve poses, breathing exercises, props, and music that cater to familiar themes, such as modes of transportation or farm animals. Despite these routines, toddler yoga classes are not rigid. Rather, the sessions are quite flexible as teachers follow the children's lead to include their interests. For example, yoga teachers may ask children to name their favorite animals and perform the corresponding poses. While mainly energetic and playful, toddler classes end with an opportunity for relaxation, which promotes calmness and self-regulation.

Classes for three- to five-year-olds

At three years of age, children typically separate from their caregivers for yoga classes as they would for preschool. This promotes independence for the child and socialization with peers. Apart from this new independence from caregivers, the structure and content of the classes for three- to five-year-old children are similar to toddler classes. They frequently include music and props, such as books, to lead children on a yoga journey. The themes and associated poses represent less familiar and more decontextualized, abstract schemas, such as underwater or outer space adventures. In addition, relaxation time at the end of the classes may include guided visualizations. Young children often exhibit difficulty lying on the floor with their eyes closed. They may fidget, open their eyes to look around, or refuse to lie down at all. Visualizations, led by a skilled yoga teacher, present children with an object of focus. These guided imaginings include various spatial, temporal, and descriptive concepts, which facilitate speech-language development in addition to mindfulness.

Classes for 5- to 12-year-olds

Yoga classes for children aged 5 to 12 years typically continue to incorporate age-appropriate music and props in addition to the poses, breathing techniques, and guided relaxations. In general, children in this age range enjoy games with rules and challenges, such as "musical mats" or "yoga jenga," rather than fantasies and stories (Cuomo 2007). Further, partner and group poses provide opportunities for socialization and communication among peers (Flynn 2013). For example, one or more children can assume "chair" pose next to or around a child in "table" pose.

Children in this age range understand increasingly complex and abstract concepts. Guided visualizations at the conclusion of classes incorporate more advanced vocabulary items. The ability to create an imagined gestalt from language serves as a basis for more sophisticated comprehension and higher-level thinking. Research indicates that the development of visual imagery improves reading and auditory comprehension, writing, expressive vocabulary, memory, and critical thinking (Bell 1991, 2007). In addition, yoga classes for school-age children support their emotional regulation and stress management.

Family classes

Family yoga classes provide opportunities for social interaction and communication across the different generations in a family. Grandparents, parents, and siblings of different ages and abilities can practice together in a positive environment. Yoga classes designed for families often emphasize group poses and games, such as family members holding hands in tree pose to create a "forest," which support bonding, confidence, and teamwork among all members. Teachers of family yoga classes are usually flexible and adapt plans to meet the needs of all participants.

Additional types of yoga classes

In the last two decades, some children's yoga classes started blending different modalities with the traditional yoga poses, breathing techniques, and meditation practices. For example, some classes combine yoga poses and breathing exercises with gymnastic activities, such as rolling and tumbling. Specifically, CircusYoga combines yoga and various circus arts, such as acrobatics and juggling, to facilitate connection, communication, and play. Another example, Glow-In-The-Dark Yoga, or GLOGA, involves children's wearing of white or neon clothing and using glow sticks, while simultaneously practicing yoga under black lights.

Some yoga classes for children emphasize the use of carefully selected children's books that naturally lead to opportunities to practice yoga while building language and literacy skills. Yoga poses and breathing exercises are incorporated into the reading of children's books, which frequently include various elements of nature, such as plants and animals. For example, yoga teachers could read the book *From Head to Toe* by Eric Carle and perform a yoga pose for each animal in the story. These unique children's yoga classes extend beyond the traditional practices to provide further opportunities to enhance the development of emergent literacy and literacy skills in children.

Classes for children with special needs

Neurodevelopmental disorders represent a group of varied conditions that involve impairment in the growth and development of the central nervous system, specifically the brain, occurring early in the developmental period (American Psychiatric Association 2013). The terms "developmental disabilities" and "special needs" are often used in clinical and educational settings to refer to individuals with these unique challenges. According to the Centers for Disease Control and Prevention (2016), approximately one in six children in the United States now present with a developmental disability. The prevalence of developmental disabilities increased 17.1 percent from 1997 to 2008, which correlates to about 1.8 million more children diagnosed with developmental disabilities. These disabilities can include impairments in cognition, communication, social skills, and adaptive functioning.

Sonia Sumar (1998) was the first yoga instructor and author to address the use of yoga with children diagnosed with developmental disabilities. Her pioneering work in yoga therapy focused on positioning and movement for the improvement of motor coordination, physical strength, and cognitive ability, first with her own daughter with Down syndrome and then primarily for other children with intellectual disabilities, cerebral palsy, learning disabilities, and attention deficit disorder (AD/HD). Sumar suggests that because yoga works on so many subsystems of the body, it can assist children with developmental disabilities to improve in the motor, cognitive, and communicative domains. While her work did not directly address the use of yoga for speech-language development, she noted improvement in her students' communication skills with the yoga practice.

Subsequently, other clinicians including Cuomo (2007), Williams (2010), Ristuccia (2010), Goldberg (2013), and

Hardy (2015), as well as other parents (e.g. Betts and Betts 2006), have written books about the benefit of yoga for children with developmental disabilities. These resources are rich in anecdotal evidence of the benefits of yoga for children with unique challenges. Of note, expert opinion is considered part of evidence-based practice (Rich 2005).

In addition, several researchers have published articles about the use of yoga with special populations. Galantino *et al.* (2008) reviewed case-control, pilot, cohort, and randomized controlled studies to investigate yoga as an exercise intervention for children, including those diagnosed with attention deficit/hyperactivity disorder (AD/HD). They found that using yoga with children as a complementary mind-body therapy produces physiological benefits during the rehabilitation process, but larger clinical trials with specific measures of quality of life are needed to provide conclusive evidence. Birdee *et al.* (2009) conducted a systematic review across pediatric and young adult populations. These investigators found that the majority of the studies revealed positive effects regarding children's physical fitness, cardiorespiratory functioning, mental health, behavior, and overall development from yoga. However, the evidence must be considered preliminary due to the methodological limitations of the reviewed studies. Serwacki and Cook-Cottone (2012) also conducted a systematic review of yoga-based interventions for various typically developing and disordered pediatric populations, including those with autism spectrum disorder (ASD), intellectual disabilities, learning impairments, and emotional disturbances. While more rigorous research designs are needed, school-based yoga programs seem beneficial for children in various ways, which include reduced stress, increased social confidence, and improved attention. Koenig *et al.* (2012) used an experimental pretest-posttest control group design to investigate the effectiveness of the "Get Ready to Learn" classroom yoga program among children with ASD. Their study revealed that the students participating in the specialized yoga program showed significantly decreased maladaptive behaviors, including irritability, lethargy, social withdrawal, hyperactivity, and noncompliance. While we recognize these numerous sensory, motor, and regulatory benefits of yoga, our emphasis in this book is on speech, language, and communication for children who are developing typically, as well as those with neurodevelopmental challenges.

Speech, language, and communication problems are prevalent as primary or secondary symptoms in all neurodevelopmental conditions. For example, children with language impairment and speech sound disorders have primary challenges in language and speech. Children with ASD present with primary impairments in communication, a core characteristic of the condition. In this book, we will address five neurodevelopmental disorders for which we believe yoga can provide an excellent complement to traditional speech-language therapy: language disorders, speech sound disorders, intellectual disabilities, ASD, and attention deficit/hyperactivity disorders (AD/HD). Of note, these conditions are not mutually exclusively and, in fact, often co-occur. For example, intellectual disability is strongly associated with a language disorder. Many, but not all, children with ASD have co-morbid intellectual disability and language impairment. The descriptions of these populations will be primarily based on the *Diagnostic and Statistical Manual of Mental Disorders, Fifth Edition* (American Psychiatric Association 2013). All of the impairments associated with these disorders must significantly impact the children's social, academic, and psychological functioning. In Chapters 4 through 9, we will infuse suggestions for the use of yoga to enhance speech, language, and communication development in children with these neurodevelopmental disorders.

Because of the limited evidence regarding yoga for speech, language, and communication, the authors of this book will present their expert clinical opinions regarding the use of yoga to facilitate development in these areas in children with neurodevelopmental challenges. They do so on the basis of their combined 55 years of experience as pediatric speech-language pathologists and 45 years as yoga practitioners. They accept full responsibility for the opinions they express.

Language disorder. A language disorder involves impairments in the comprehension and/or production of language (American Psychiatric Association 2013) in form, content, and/or use (Lahey 1988), domains which were introduced in Chapter 2. These impairments must be distinguished from language differences, which include dialectal variations and limited exposure due to second language learning (Pence Turnbull and Justice 2017). Children with language impairments can demonstrate reduced word and sentence structure (the form of language), vocabulary and concepts (the content of language), and/or conversational and narrative skills (the use of language). These impairments are considered primary in the absence of any other developmental challenges, such as hearing loss, motor dysfunction, intellectual disability, or other neurological conditions (American Psychiatric Association 2013; Pence Turnbull and Justice 2017). Once it is established that these children are not merely "late talkers," they are diagnosed with "specific language impairment" (SLI), a term commonly used by speech-language pathologists (Leonard 2014; Pence Turnbull and Justice 2017) to refer to this population. The prevalence of SLI for kindergartners in the upper Midwestern region of the United States was 7.4 percent overall (Tomblin *et al.* 1997). Language impairments also exist *secondary* to other conditions, such as intellectual disability and ASD (Pence Turnbull and Justice 2017), which will be subsequently described.

Speech sound disorder. Speech sound disorder is an umbrella term relating to difficulties with the perception, articulation, and/or phonological representation of speech sounds and segments. The errors include phoneme (speech sound) additions, omissions, distortions, or substitutions (American Psychiatric Association 2013). These misarticulations interfere with the intelligibility of children's speech and the listener's ability to understand their verbal messages. Speech sound disorders are often diagnosed when speech sound production is below expectations for age and developmental level. By age four, children's speech should be fully intelligible (Coplan and Gleason 1988; Flipsen 2006). Speech sound disorders can be motor-based as in apraxia and dysarthria, structurally based as in cleft palate and other craniofacial anomalies, syndrome/condition-related as in Down syndrome and metabolic conditions (e.g. galactosemia), and sensory-based as in hearing impairment. The most widely cited summary of speech sound disorder prevalence is based on a systematic review conducted by Law *et al.* (2000), who reported that 2 percent to 25 percent of children aged five to seven years have this challenge. More recent prevalence data suggests that 8 percent to 9 percent of children have speech sound disorders (National Institute on Deafness and Other Communication Disorders 2010).

Intellectual disability. Intellectual disability is characterized by clinically significant impairments in two areas, namely intellectual ability and adaptive functioning. Manifestations of intellectual impairment include challenges in reasoning, problem solving, abstract thinking, judgment, and experiential learning. Adaptive functioning refers to the level of personal independence and social responsibility that is expected for an individual's age and cultural group. Adaptive behaviors are important across different environments including home, school, and community (American Psychiatric Association 2013). All individuals in this population have a speech-language-communication impairment that is secondary to their intellectual disability (Pence Turnbull and Justice 2017). According to the Centers for Disease Control and Prevention (2016), 12 in 1000 children exhibit mild to severe intellectual disability. This indicates that intellectual disability occurs in approximately 1 percent of the general population (American Psychiatric Association 2013).

Autism spectrum disorder. ASD refers to a broad category of neurodevelopmental disabilities defined by two core characteristics, namely 1) impairments in social communication and social interaction and 2) the presence of restricted, repetitive patterns of behaviors, interests, and activities (American Psychiatric Association 2013). Deficits in both of these areas must be present in order for an individual to be diagnosed with ASD. Although the onset of the condition must occur in the early developmental period, usually before three years, symptoms might not be manifest until somewhat later when the demands of social communication exceed the child's capacities. ASD has increased in prevalence over the past two decades, perhaps due to a widening of the spectrum to include milder cases, increased awareness of the early signs of the disability, a combination of the two, or some other factor. Current estimates of the prevalence of ASD are 1 in 68 (Centers for Disease Control and Prevention 2016).

Attention deficit/hyperactivity disorder. Attention deficit/hyperactivity disorder (AD/HD) refers to a persistent pattern of inattention and/or hyperactivity/impulsivity that interferes with an individual's functioning or development (American Psychiatric Association 2013). Challenges manifest in areas such as sustaining attention to an activity, following directions, engaging in sequential tasks, and being easily distracted by environmental stimuli. Children with hyperactivity engage in impulsive behaviors such as fidgeting at a level that is inconsistent with their developmental level, show difficulty waiting for their turn, and often move during inappropriate times. Estimates of AD/HD vary from about 5 percent (American Psychiatric Association 2013) to 11 percent of the pediatric population (Centers for Disease Control and Prevention 2016).

Due to the rise in the number of children with these neurodevelopmental disabilities, additional health and education services are needed (Boyle *et al.* 2011). Fortunately, yoga classes for children with special needs are becoming increasingly available. Group yoga classes promote communication and socialization opportunities among peers for these special populations. For example, a child with ASD who presents with social challenges may benefit from stretching with a peer during a group class. In contrast, private sessions provide opportunities for one-to-one interactions between the child and yoga instructor and are appropriate for children with unique challenges that may not be addressed in a group setting. These individualized classes accommodate individual preferences, strengths, limitations, and learning styles to help children from special populations meet their developmental goals and improve overall functioning. For example, a child with AD/HD who may be distracted by the use of props and the presence of other children may benefit from individual instruction. Families of children with developmental disabilities and yoga teachers can form partnerships to determine whether group or private classes are appropriate to best meet individual needs and facilitate all areas of development (Goldberg 2013), including speech, language, and communication.

Trends in children's yoga classes

While the structure and content of children's yoga classes vary depending on the setting, teacher, age range, and developmental level, several commonalities exist. Most children's yoga classes incorporate a variety of appropriate materials, including recorded music, musical instruments, art supplies, books, puppets, and other toys to help children participate in yoga practices. Some classes allow children to bring their favorite doll or stuffed animal to practice alongside them on miniature yoga mats. Beginning playfully and energetically, children's yoga classes typically conclude with relaxation. This relaxation time for children often involves specific activities, such as foot massages from instructors or caregivers to provide tactile input, aromatherapy (with essential oils) to harmonize the body, and guided visualizations to expand imagination.

Most importantly, children's yoga classes focus on enjoyment and exploration rather than proper alignment and breath coordination. Optimal learning occurs in conjunction with positive emotional states (Willis 2006). The light, playful nature of children's yoga classes evokes these positive emotions, and consequently facilitates brain development, especially long-term memory of learned skills.

Summary

The literature, while limited, suggests that yoga helps children in the physical, cognitive, and social-emotional domains. Because of its growing popularity and emerging evidence-base, yoga classes can be increasingly found in local communities for infants and their caregivers, toddlers, preschoolers, school-age children, and families. Yoga classes can be conducted on an individual or group basis in a variety of settings—at home, in yoga studios, community centers, and schools. Both typically developing children and children with a variety of neurodevelopmental conditions including language disorders, speech sound disorders, intellectual disability, ASD, and attention deficit/hyperactivity disorder (AD/HD) can enjoy and benefit from yoga sessions or classes. For children with these latter challenges, yoga can complement traditional forms of speech-language therapy conducted by a knowledgeable yoga practitioner/clinician.

PART II

YOGA FOR DIFFERENT DEVELOPMENTAL DOMAINS

Chapter 4

YOGA FOR PRELINGUISTIC COMMUNICATION

In order to develop normally, a child requires progressively more complex joint activity with one or more adults who have an irrational emotional relationship with the child. Somebody's got to be crazy about that kid. That's number one. First, last, and always.

Urie Bronfenbrenner

Introduction to prelinguistic communication

Communication is the process of sharing information among individuals. As introduced in Chapter 2, the prelinguistic stage of language development can be subdivided into the preintentional and intentional stages. In the first preintentional stage, which lasts from birth to about eight months, adults frequently interpret babies' behaviors such as smiling or crying as if they were purposeful, intentional acts before infants have actually developed the capacity to communicate intentionally, which emerges at about seven to eight months. In order to understand infants' prelinguistic development, their concurrent social-emotional growth must be considered. Greenspan's (1985) model of the stages of social-emotional development provides a useful theoretical framework in which the stages of language development can be considered in broader developmental perspectives. He noted that during the earliest months from birth to about three months, infants focus on the challenge of self-regulation and use their senses to develop interest in the world around them. Following this initial period, up to about seven months, infants focus on forming relationships with their caregivers and engaging in affective vocal synchrony with them. These two stages map onto the preintentional stage of language development. In the second half of the first year, infants enter the intentional stage of language development with the prelinguistic child engaging in purposeful, two-way communication as its hallmark. In Greenspan's (1985) model of social-emotional development, intentional two-way communication at 8 to 12 months is key.

Prelinguistic communication refers to the infant's intentional engagement with another through nonlinguistic means, namely gestures, gaze, and vocalizations. Infants often use these prelinguistic forms of communication in combination with one another. For example, a baby might gaze and vocalize or gesture at his caregiver or produce all three prelinguistic forms of communication simultaneously. In this way, infants can communicate a variety of intentions such as expressing feelings and sharing in joint action routines. These prelinguistic forms and functions of communication are evident before the emergence of first words, which was discussed in Chapter 2. Further as noted in Chapter 3, yoga classes for infants and their caregivers provide a context for facilitating prelinguistic communication skills, such as eye gaze, shared attention, and turn-taking, which are manifestations of the infants' engagement with their caregivers. A challenge with engagement with others is a core feature of autism spectrum disorders (ASD) (American Psychiatric Association 2013) and a characteristic of several other clinical populations. In addition, caregiver-baby yoga at the prelinguistic stage, as well as yoga classes for children in the later stages of language development, fosters the comprehension of language in the context of simple routines.

Yoga and prelinguistic communication

Yoga can enhance prelinguistic communication for infants who range in age from approximately six weeks to one year. Whether led in a group class under the watchful eye of a skilled instructor or conducted in the convenience of the home, yoga practices for this age group allow mothers and other caregivers to bond more deeply with their babies through various senses including the tactile, visual, and auditory as well as through coordinated rhythm of the breath cycle, which will be discussed in Chapter 5. For parents and newborns, bonding, which refers to awareness of the relationship between one's self and another person, can take place through "a shared steady gaze" (Garabedian 2004, p.41). Garabedian notes that yoga facilitates caregivers' responsiveness to "their child's intentions, needs, and desires" (Garabedian 2004, p.ix), factors related to language development. In addition to facilitating bonding and prelinguistic development, yoga exercises for infants help foster neuromuscular development, digestion, circulation, and sleep (Garabedian 2004; Larson and Howard 2002).

Eye gaze

Within a few short weeks following birth, at about seven weeks, infants spend increased amounts of time gazing at the human face because they find that several of its aspects are compelling (Stern 1985). The curves of the cheeks and eyebrows, the angles of the corners of the eyes, the contrast of the darkness of the pupils with the lightness of the rest of the eyes, the symmetry of the two sides of the face, and the motion of talking mouths all fascinate infants. In essence, preintentional infants can appear riveted by faces. Babies' gaze at others, also called eye contact, reflects their engagement with the adults in their environment. In caregiver-baby yoga, the baby is always positioned comfortably in close physical proximity to his caregiver. Sometimes the baby lies next to or in front of the adult on a small blanket or towel.

At other times, the baby rests directly on his caregiver's body. The optimal positions to facilitate engagement, communication, and speech-language development occur when the baby faces the adult (Pepper and Weitzman 2004). When caregiver and child face one another, the infant has the opportunity both to initiate interaction and to respond to adult-initiated interaction, paving the groundwork for later conversations. When the baby enters into these dialogues with his parents or another caregiver (Greenspan 1985), the adult can talk to the baby about the ongoing action of the yoga routine or sing rhymes or songs that accompany the movement. Garabedian (2004, p.17) provides many examples of this "Sing and Do" technique, in which the adult uses a "slow and melodic speaking voice" to accompany the yoga movements. Speech-language pathologists refer to this type of speech register as infant-directed or child-directed speech, which has replaced the formerly used terms "motherese" or "parentese" in the professional literature (Newman and Sachs 2017). Another characteristic of this speech input is that it codes the "here and now" of the ongoing moment. Garabedian (2004, p.17) suggests singing "toes to nose" as caregivers perform the action of bringing their baby's toes to their nose and then tickling their baby's nose with their toes in a playful fashion. In this way, the caregiver's talk coordinates the movement with linguistic input, supporting the child's comprehension. Larson and Howard (2002) similarly provide specific suggestions of songs such as "Open, Shut Them" and rhymes that could be used in this way.

As noted in the previous chapter, massage is sometimes incorporated into yoga classes for children. In yoga classes for infants, a gentle baby massage is often used as part of a session. Whether done as part of a group yoga class or at other times such as right before or after a bath at home, massage is an excellent tool to foster the caregiver's bonding with her baby (Garabedian 2004; Larson and Howard 2002). As baby massage is always conducted with the child lying supine looking up, this activity can also facilitate engagement.

During the massage, the caregivers can produce infant-directed speech as they label their child's body parts from head to toes while they administer gentle strokes with open palms. Garabedian (2004) describes a massage-like technique, which she calls "Heart-Warm Touch." In this practice, the infant lies on his back while facing the caregiver who vigorously rubs her hands together creating heat. Then the caregiver gently massages her infant from shoulders to toes while imagining that her heart is glowing. This activity was designed to soothe both caregiver and baby.

Infant massage as part of a yoga practice can be initiated with newborns and adapted as infants and toddlers develop in the physical, emotional, and linguistic domains. An option for linguistic input that accompanies massage for infants who are about six weeks or older is to engage in an adapted counting game such as "one yoga-sippi, two yoga-sippi, three yoga-sippi," up to ten as caregivers administer long, gentle strokes from head to toes over the entire length of their baby's body. As it is easier to massage babies before they are six months, this practice is ideally suited for the preintentional child. In addition to engagement, the soothing nature of massage as sensory input assists the baby in attaining a calm, regulated state, which is consistent with Greenspan's (1985) first developmental stage mentioned earlier.

Obtaining a calm, regulated state is a challenge for some children with neurodevelopmental disabilities, including children with ASD and attention deficit/hyperactivity disorder (AD/HD). Children from these populations may benefit from the soothing, deep pressure massage. Sumar (1998) provides specific procedures for using infant massage with children with Down syndrome and other special populations. She notes that massage facilitates relaxation, stimulates blood flow, and provides a context for caregiver/child bonding. Like Larson and Howard (2002), she recommends that the adult incorporate the names of the body parts into the activity.

In terms of yoga poses, several, including boat, bound angle, bridge, cobra, sphinx, and cat, are well suited for face-to-face interaction, providing a context for the baby's engagement with their caregiver.

In boat pose (Figure 4.1a), the caregiver is seated on the floor and the infant is positioned in the crook of the adult's legs. The adult can sing "Row, Row, Row Your Boat" while holding the baby's hands, which can be moved like oars. The repetitive, rhythmical lyrics, coordinated with the movement, provide a joint action routine for the caregiver-child social partners, what Bruner (1983) called "formats," which were introduced in Chapter 2. In addition, the baby can lie prone on his caregiver's lower legs while the caregiver holds both of the infant's hands. Caregivers can then extend their legs into a more challenging boat pose while the baby moves up and down. During this joint action routine, the caregiver can say "elevator up" or simply "up" and "elevator down" or simply "down," timing their linguistic input with the baby's up and down movements which facilitates language comprehension. "Bumpin' Up and Down," a song popularized by Raffi, could also be used in this context (Larson and Howard 2002).

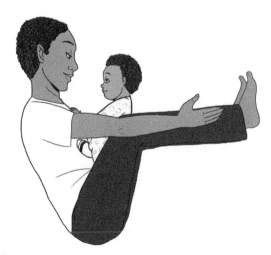

Figure 4.1a Boat pose

In bound angle pose (Figure 4.1b), the adult is also seated on the floor, but the baby's head rests face up near the caregiver's feet. The adult can vocalize, sing, or otherwise talk to the baby providing infant-directed speech. For example, the adult can lean in toward the baby while saying "hello" or his name. In addition, as the adult's hands are free in this pose, she can cover then expose her eyes to play "peek-a-boo" with her baby. This can provide a highly engaging context for prelinguistic communication.

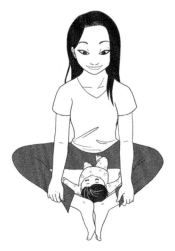

Figure 4.1b Bound angle pose

In bridge pose (Figure 4.1c), the adult lies on her back with knees bent and feet flat on the floor, then raises and lowers her pelvis while the baby sits on her abdomen, which lifts the baby up and down. The caregiver can add fun words such as "whee" which, like the chant "om," provides maximal labial contrast. In the syllable "whee" the lips move from a rounded posture for the consonant /w/ to a spread lip position for the vowel "ee" written phonetically as /i/. For the production of "om," the lips move from the rounded vowel position for /OU/ to the bilabial closed position for the consonant "m" written phonetically as /m/.

In addition, the caregiver could produce the monosyllabic locative action terms "up" and "down" simultaneously with the movement, exposing the child to these early words.

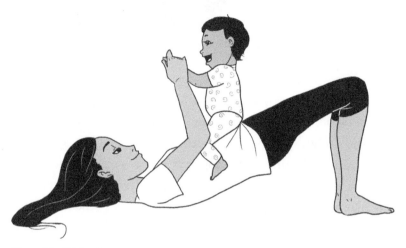

Figure 4.1c Bridge pose

Cobra pose (Figure 4.1d) provides another opportunity for the caregiver and her infant to be positioned face-to-face. In cobra, the caregiver lies prone on her abdomen with her legs extended straight behind her, tops of the feet flat on the floor, arms bent with hands touching the floor beneath the shoulders. In sphinx pose, which is similar to cobra, the caregiver lies prone on her abdomen with her legs in the same position as cobra, but her arms are bent at the elbows with her forearms touching the floor beneath the shoulders. In both cobra and sphinx, the baby can lie on a folded blanket on the caregiver's mat at the level of her shoulders or be seated in front of her if able to do so unassisted. In either position, the baby can gaze at the mother and reach toward her face. In cobra, the caregiver can produce a prolonged /s/ sound with teeth together and lips spread into a smile to mimic the sound of a snake. Appropriate infant-directed speech such as "I see you!" can be added to either pose.

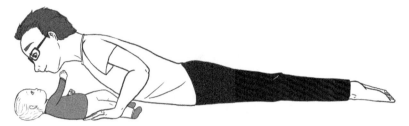

Figure 4.1d Cobra pose

Cat-cow poses also provide an excellent opportunity for face-to-face interaction, responsiveness, and lexical stimulation. In these poses the caregiver begins by kneeling on all fours in a neutral spine position forming a tabletop with hands directly under the shoulders and knees directly below the hips. The infant lies supine on a blanket facing up toward the caregiver. As the caregiver moves into an arched spinal posture for cow, she can make a mooing sound mimicking a cow. As she moves into a rounded spinal posture for cat, she can make the meowing sound of a cat or provide some other appropriate speech input (Figure 4.1e). In addition, the caregiver can smile and shake her head from side to side, letting her hair fly, which the baby will enjoy (Larson and Howard 2002). In the same beginning neutral posture on all fours as in cat-cow, the caregiver can "wag the tail." In this variation the caregiver looks over each shoulder moving her head from side to side. When the head crosses midline, she can smile, vocalize, or otherwise engage the baby who is lying supine face up.

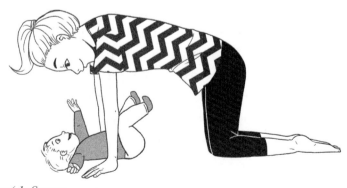

Figure 4.1e Cat pose

Reciprocity

While in boat, bound angle, bridge, cobra, sphinx, or other face-to-face poses, the caregiver can produce monosyllabic vowel-consonant (VC) syllables which might be chants, such as "om," while the baby watches her mouth move from the open position for the vowel to the bilabial closed lip posture for the consonant. Other VC or CV syllables which could be simple chants or nonsense syllables can be used in this context. The infant could be encouraged to vocalize in alternation or in unison with the caregiver. Vocalizing in alternation involves turn-taking or reciprocity between the communicative partners on a prelinguistic level. These vocal behaviors provide a foundation for later speech development. When the caregiver sings songs, the child can vocalize or produce a movement as if taking a turn. For example, the baby can vocalize or move his arms with adult assistance during the song that begins "Wind, wind, wind them [say baby's name]" described in Larson and Howard (2002). Songs such as "Hop Along Yogi" and "Yogi, Yogi" adapted from the familiar "Hokey Pokey" (Garabedian 2004) provide opportunities for reciprocal interaction. These songs could facilitate reciprocity between children with ASD and their caregivers, as challenges in social interaction are a core characteristic of their disability. Once the songs become an established routine, their repetition will help foster interaction as it is well established that children with ASD learn best in predictable contexts.

Gestures

Gestures are actions that are produced with the intent to communicate (Crais, Douglas, and Campbell 2004). These actions are typically produced through fingers, hands, and arms, but can also include facial features and body movements. Deictic gestures call attention to or indicate an object or event, such as reaching toward or pointing to the mother's face. The most commonly studied deictic gestures in infants are showing, giving, reaching, and pointing, which develop with the emergence of intentionality at around eight months. Impaired use of gestures to express these intentions is another manifestation of the core deficit in social interaction of young children with ASD.

After deictic gestures are used to signal objects, people, or events in the environment, they are used to signal shared or joint attention to an object or event. This requires that the infant coordinate attention to an object or event with a social partner. A lack of joint attention in infancy is an indication of the social communication deficit in ASD and an early recognized red flag for this developmental disability. In addition, some children with AD/HD are so busy that they have difficulty sustaining attention for joint attention and turn-taking activities. Joint attention is an important communication developmental milestone, which emerges in the intentional prelinguistic period, and is a prerequisite to conversations (Pence Turnbull and Justice 2017), in which topics become a shared focus between speakers. In caregiver-baby yoga, the adult is the social partner and the movement, sounds, or words become the object or event of focus. For example, in the joint action routine that accompanies the song "Hop Along Yogi" (Garabedian 2004), the baby's turns consist of slow or fast and up or down actions caused by the caregiver's leg movements.

Another type of gesture, called "representational" (Crais *et al.* 2004), indicates or represents something. This type of gesture is also challenging for children with ASD. For example, in a common caregiver-infant routine, the adult asks, "How big is the baby?" and the baby lifts his arms upward, indicating "so big." In addition to providing an opportunity for reciprocity and the facilitation of language comprehension of the lexical item "big," lifting the baby's arms in this routine to produce the representational gesture has the added benefit of expanding the baby's chest, which facilitates breath support for speech, an area of challenge for children with Down syndrome who have low muscle tone and poor trunk stability. The topic of breath support for speech will be discussed in Chapter 5.

Comprehension

During the prelinguistic stage of language development, before infants have begun to talk, most children begin to comprehend language. Comprehension refers to the ability to understand what others say. The repetition and predictability of objects, events, and movements in everyday routines paired with language help facilitate young children's comprehension. Children with language disorders can be impaired in both their comprehension and production of language, although many children with language impairments, like typically developing children, have relatively better receptive than expressive language. However, the language patterns of children with ASD often do not conform to this pattern. Their comprehension problems can be greater than their expressive impairments (American Psychiatric Association 2013).

The context of a baby massage, which was described earlier, provides an opportunity to facilitate language comprehension. In this context, the baby hears his name and the names of various body parts. When engaged in yoga with their caregivers at home or in a "Mommy and Me" type of class, infants can learn the names of some body parts, simple actions, locations, and directions, referred to as one-step commands. For example, while lying on their backs face-to-face with their caregivers, infants can hear the rhyming words "toes to nose". Infants can be instructed to "touch your toes" or "open and close" arms or legs while performing these actions with adult facilitation. Adult facilitated infant leg movements for flexion and extension can be accompanied by the locative action words "in" and "out." The adult can also facilitate infant torso twisting or rolling movements to each side using directional words such as "left and right" or "back and forth" or the verbs "twisting" or "rolling" as the appropriate movement is performed. As noted previously, the caregiver can add the words "up" and "down" to appropriate movements such as in bridge pose, fostering comprehension of these locative action terms. Similarly, the child will hear the descriptive terms "fast" and "slow" while participating in the "Hop Along Yogi" routine mentioned above, facilitating the comprehension of those words. The classes can also provide a context for the baby to hear his name as the instructor refers to the various caregiver-child dyads. At home, the caregiver can also sing the child's name in face-to-face interaction in a variety of everyday contexts to facilitate comprehension of this important term. Garabedian suggests a variation of the "Hop Along Yogi" song (Garabedian 2004) in which the baby's name replaces the word "yogi." This adaptation could work with other songs and routines. The foregoing suggestions apply to all children, those who are typically developing and those who are neurodevelopmentally impaired.

Books and other resources

Speech-language pathologists are familiar with the importance of engaging in shared book reading with prelinguistic children (Pepper and Weitzman 2004). However, developmentally young children need active learning experiences and cannot learn to practice yoga through books! Nevertheless, books can serve as a context for joint attention and for providing the baby with early emergent literacy experiences. The topic of emergent literacy will be explored in Chapter 9. In terms of specific children's books, we did not identify any with a yogic orientation that were specifically for infants, but several were written for toddlers in the second year of life and the early preschool years. One notable yoga book that is geared for toddlers and the early preschool years that could be adapted and read to prelinguistic infants, especially those who are intentional, is Rebecca Whitford's *Little Yoga: A Toddler's First Book of Yoga*.

Summary

Caregiver-baby yoga practiced from about six weeks until the end of the first year or when the baby becomes an independent walker provides a context for prelinguistic development for both the preintentional and intentional infant as well as for children with neurodevelopmental challenges who are functioning at this very early stage of speech-language development. In addition to the benefits for the post-pregnancy mother in terms of returning to her pre-pregnancy physical condition, she and the baby's other caretakers will have an opportunity to bond with the baby through the various poses, songs, rhymes, and other practices described in this chapter. In addition, the preintentional infant will have an opportunity to engage with their caretaker in the context of the baby yoga practice. The intentional prelinguistic child will be able to practice some gestures and turn-taking while engaging with his caregiver in yoga. Finally, the infant will be exposed to language in the context of the predictability and repetitiveness of the yoga routines, which will map words to meaning to aid comprehension. All of this happens while both caregivers and their children share special time together. The resource tables in Appendices 2–8 of this book contain information on yoga books, card decks, games, CDs, DVDs, and websites to enhance prelinguistic communication development in children.

Chapter 5

YOGA FOR BREATH SUPPORT FOR SPEECH

Breath is the link between mind and body.

Dan Brulé

Introduction to respiration

The process of respiration involves the exchange of gas between an organism and its environment (Seikel, King, and Drumright 2000). In humans, respiration, also known as breathing, is subdivided into the processes of inspiration and expiration. Through the process of inspiration, humans inhale which brings oxygen to the cells of the body. Through the process of expiration, humans exhale which releases carbon dioxide from the body. The lungs, the major paired organs of respiration, contain no skeletal muscles of their own to power this movement. Consequently, the work of breathing is performed by the surrounding musculature. Depending on the needs of the body, quiet inspiration involves only the diaphragm, a large dome-shaped muscle that separates the thoracic and abdominal cavities. When the diaphragm contracts and descends during the inhalation phase of breathing, the volume of the thoracic cavity increases, and the air pressure inside the cavity concomitantly decreases. In this state, the air pressure inside the lungs is lower than atmospheric pressure.

Consequently, air enters the lungs until the two pressures equalize (Seikel *et al.* 2000).

In contrast to quiet inspiration, forced inspiration requires the activation of the external intercostal muscles, which are located between the 12 pairs of ribs in the thoracic cavity. These muscles provide mobility and unity to the rib cage. The external intercostal muscles are considered accessory muscles because inspiration can occur without them. However, by elevating the rib cage, the external intercostal muscles significantly increase the quantity of air inhaled into the lungs. Other accessory muscles that contribute to forced inspiration reside in the thorax, as well as in the neck, shoulder, and arm regions of the body (Seikel *et al.* 2000).

During quiet expiration, the diaphragm relaxes and ascends, decreasing the volume of the thoracic cavity and concomitantly increasing air pressure. Consequently, air flows out of the body until the pressure between the lungs and the atmosphere equalizes. Three passive forces, namely torque, elasticity, and gravity, drive the exhalation phase of breathing by restoring the respiratory system to a resting position. First, torque, the rotary restoration force, unwinds the cartilages adjacent to the sternum that twist and elevate during inspiration. Second, the porous, highly elastic nature of lung tissue, which stretches during inspiration, facilitates return of the lungs to their original size and shape. Third, gravity pulls the ribs back to rest in both standing and sitting positions (Seikel *et al.* 2000).

In contrast to quiet expiration, forced expiration requires musculature to act indirectly on the lungs to "squeeze" air out of them. As the rib cage is elevated during inspiration, the internal intercostal muscles, the innermost layer of the intercostals, and the transverse thoracic muscles are activated to depress the rib cage. In addition, several abdominal muscles contract to compress the abdomen and move the internal organs, such as the intestines, in an upward direction. This reduces the size of the thorax (Seikel *et al.* 2000). Figure 5.1 illustrates the two processes of inspiration (inhalation) and expiration (exhalation) that comprise respiration.

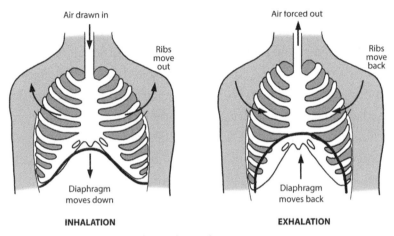

Figure 5.1 Inhalation and exhalation phases of respiration

Respiration for speech production

Differences exist between non-speech and speech breathing. Speech involves the movement and coordination of the respiratory, phonatory, resonatory, and articulatory systems. Respiration, which sustains life itself, is the foundation of the four systems that are involved in speech production. For the inhalation phase of respiration, non-speech breathing generally involves more reflexive, less conscious control, whereas speech breathing involves more voluntary, conscious control (Tobey and Rampp 1987). During speech breathing, the speaker needs to increase the quantity of air inhaled in order to have sufficient breath capacity to complete an utterance without interruption. This could be achieved by increasing either the depth or duration of inhalation, or both. For exhalation, a relatively constant supply of air pressure below the vocal folds is needed to drive phonation. The respiratory system can quickly and momentarily change this pressure to adapt to the linguistic demands of an utterance, such as syllable stress (Seikel *et al.* 2000).

Development of speech breathing in children

Similar to the development of other motor skills, the development of speech breathing progresses through periods of emergence and refinement (Boliek *et al.* 2009). The emergence period, which occurs from birth to three years of age, involves gradual changes in speech breathing that relate to anatomical, neurological, and biomechanical growth. For example, an increase in the size of the lungs results in increased air volumes used during speech breathing. However, like all aspects of early development, this emergence period is characterized by variability, such as the duration of the exhalation phase of breathing. During the refinement period of speech breathing, the respiratory system continues to grow as the length and complexity of spoken utterances increases. Breath support for speech continues to develop into adolescence (Hixon and Hoit 2005) allowing for increased vocal intensity, improved speech intelligibility, and the production of a greater number of words per minute (Wills, Seberg, and Economides 2014).

Benefits of yoga breathwork for speech production

As discussed in Chapter 1, conscious breathing is one of the three main practices in yoga. Yoga enables children to increase their awareness or become mindful of the breath. Long, deep inhalations and exhalations increase oxygen supply and eliminate toxins, which the body needs to do to function properly.

The consistent practice of yoga poses strengthens and elongates muscles, especially those located in the trunk (specifically, the neck, chest, abdomen, and pelvis) in order to maintain proper alignment for efficient breathing. As all movements develop in a proximal (the spine) to distal (the extremities) direction, a strong trunk is necessary to produce the fine motor movements of the jaw, lips, and tongue needed for articulate speech (Wills 2015).

Down syndrome is a congenital disorder resulting from an extra chromosome, which causes intellectual disabilities, language delays, physical abnormalities, and various health issues. Children with Down syndrome typically present with low muscle tone throughout their body, including the trunk. Muscle tone refers to the resting length of muscles in the body. In low muscle tone, the resting length of the muscles is greater than average as in children with Down syndrome. While congenital low muscle tone cannot be changed, yoga poses and breathwork can strengthen muscles, resulting in decreased effects of low muscle tone and increased trunk stability. This stability leads to improved alignment, respiration, and speech production.

Breathwork for the infant years

As explained in Chapter 3, the infant's participation in yoga is relatively passive, whereas the caregiver's role is active. In order to try to synchronize breathing, an adult can place one hand on her own chest and her other hand on the baby's chest. Similarly, the caregiver can lay the baby on her chest to encourage synchronization of their breathing cycles. These acts could initiate the process of increasing the child's awareness of the breath.

Breathwork for the toddler and preschool years

As discussed in Chapter 3, a child becomes an active yoga participant when his walking skills have become more firmly established around 18 to 24 months. In order to continue to increase the young child's awareness of the breath, as well as begin to control the flow of air in and out of the body, it is beneficial to provide auditory, verbal, visual, tactile, and kinesthetic feedback regarding the adult and the child's performance of various breathing exercises. The following activities can be performed with toddlers and preschool-age children with adult facilitation either on an individual basis or in a group setting. Children with attention deficit/hyperactivity disorder (AD/HD) should particularly benefit from the sustained attention to the breath.

- *Listening breath.* The child cups his hands over his ears so that he can hear the breath (Simpkins and Simpkins 2011).

- *Blowing breath.* The child blows bubbles or pinwheels so that he can see the effect of the exhalation.

- *Three-part breath.* The child places his hands sequentially on his chest, ribs, and abdomen in order to feel the movements associated with each of these three areas of respiration.

- *Belly breath.* When the child lies down, an adult places a soft toy on his abdomen and instructs him to use the breath to move the toy gently up and down without it falling off his body. For example, the adult places a rubber duck on the child's abdomen and tells him to make "waves" by breathing in and out of the belly while watching the duck "swim." This activity allows the child to see the movement caused by the breath. This could be particularly helpful to children with intellectual disabilities and autism spectrum disorder (ASD) as it provides a concrete, external sign of the internal process of respiration. Figure 5.2 illustrates a boy practicing belly breath.

- *Spherical breath.* A Hoberman sphere is a children's toy that resembles a geodesic dome; it expands and contracts by the scissor-like action of its joints. The child holds a Hoberman sphere in his hands. As the child inhales and moves his hands apart, the sphere grows bigger. As he exhales and moves his hands together, the dome grows smaller (Rawlinson 2013). This visual-motor activity can facilitate an increase in the duration and volume of the breath. Using the sphere could be beneficial for children with AD/HD as it provides a concrete object to manipulate and may help them sustain attention. For children with intellectual disabilities and ASD, the sphere could provide a concrete, external representation of the process of respiration.

- *Counting breath.* The adult and/or child counts the duration of the inhalations and exhalations. This count should increase over time reflecting strengthened respiratory control (Simpkins and Simpkins 2011).

- *Color breath.* The adult or child assigns different colors for inhalations and exhalations (e.g. yellow for inhalation and blue for exhalation) so that the child can visualize and maintain attention to the breath (Simpkins and Simpkins 2011).

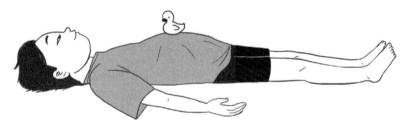

Figure 5.2 Belly breath

The subsequent breathing activities involve an aspect of symbolic play, which will be addressed in Chapter 8. In these activities, the child represents animals or objects by using their breath in conjunction with other parts of the body. Due to their difficulty with pretend play, these breathing activities can be particularly beneficial for children with ASD. For children from this population, using a picture symbol for the animals and objects named in the breathing exercises could facilitate their ability to comprehend them.

- *Bunny breath.* The child keeps his chin down as he takes three quick "sniffs" followed by a long exhalation through the nose (Rawlinson 2013).

- *Bee breath.* The child first inhales deeply and then creates a long "humming" exhalation (Rawlinson 2013). The child can make high- and low-pitched humming sounds in order to hear the differences in the frequencies of the two types of sounds. It is important for the child's face and lips to remain relaxed so that he can also feel the different types of vibrations generated from the high- and low-pitched sounds.

- *Snake breath.* The child inhales deeply and "hisses" slowly by prolonging the production of the /s/ sound on the exhalation.

- *Candle breath.* The child joins the palms of the hands in front of him pretending to form a candle. The child inhales through the nose and exhales through the mouth in order to blow out the imaginary flame.

- *Flower breath.* The child holds an actual flower or pretends to hold an imaginary one. The child inhales through the nose and prolongs the vocalization "ah" on the exhalation.

- *Whale breath.* The child first inhales through the nose and then tilts his head back to exhale through a "blowhole" made with cupped hands. Figure 6.3 in the next chapter illustrates a boy practicing whale breath.

- *Elephant breath.* The child stands with his feet apart, interlaces his hands, and allows his arms to dangle in front of him like an elephant's trunk. The child inhales through the nose as he raises his arms and exhales through the mouth as he swings his arms down through his legs. Figure 5.3 illustrates a girl practicing elephant breath.

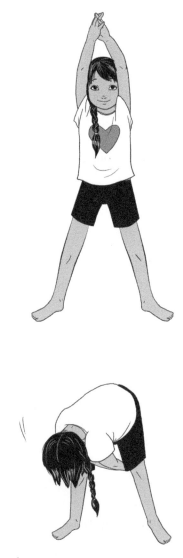

Figure 5.3 Elephant breath

All of these breathing activities increase the child's awareness of the breath, as well as facilitate learning to differentially control the inhalation and the exhalation phases of the breathing cycle.

Breathwork for the school-age years

As mentioned in Chapter 3, children of five years of age and older generally prefer exercises and activities with rules and challenges rather than ones that are primarily symbolic. In addition, school-age children understand increasingly complex and abstract language concepts (Nippold 2007). Therefore, breathing exercises can involve the comprehension of directions with more advanced spatial, temporal, and descriptive terms. The following breathing exercises, which can be performed with fading adult facilitation to promote independence, aid the development of further control over the respiratory system in order to enhance breath support for speech.

- *Hand cooling breath.* The child purses his lips and blows into the palm of his hand so that it feels cool and dry (Goldberg 2013).

- *Hand warming breath.* The child opens his mouth and exhales into the palm of his hand so that it feels warm and moist (Goldberg 2013).

- *Breath of fire.* The child inhales and exhales vigorously through the nose; as a result, the abdomen moves in and out rapidly.

- *Alternate nostril breath.* The child brings the right hand in front of his face with the thumb adjacent to the right nostril and the ring finger adjacent to the left nostril. First the child closes the right nostril with the thumb and inhales through the left nostril. Then the child closes the left nostril with the ring finger and exhales through the right nostril. Last the child inhales through the right nostril, closes the right nostril with the thumb, and exhales through the left nostril. This sequence completes one round of alternate nostril breathing.

- *Langhana breath.* The child's exhalation is twice the duration of the inhalation. For example, the child inhales for a count of two, then exhales for a count of four. The count can be adjusted according to the needs of the child.

- *Mountain breath.* Using paper and a writing instrument, the child can draw his breath. As the child inhales, he draws an upward line, and as the child exhales, he draws a downward line in order to create hills or mountains with the breath.

- *Nature breath.* The child connects the breath to elements of nature, such as the sounds of the ocean by inhaling as the waves roll into the beach and exhaling as the waves roll out to sea.

- *Smile chant.* For the smile chant, the child first inhales and then produces the vowel "e," phonetically represented as /i/, on the exhalation. Gradually, the child prolongs the "e" on the exhalation, which facilitates breath support for speech (Goldberg 2013).

- *Mantra breath.* The child uses a mantra, which is a sound, syllable, word, phrase, or sentence repeated to aid concentration, while engaging in breathing exercises. For example, the child can inhale while thinking "I am" and exhale while thinking "strong." To improve confidence regarding communication skills, the child can use the mantras "I can speak" or "I talk well" during breathing activities.

All of the foregoing breathing exercises, which provide a point of focus, can assist children with AD/HD to sustain attention.

Furthermore, as school-age children typically enjoy group activities, breathing exercises can be performed with one or more partners. For example, by sitting back-to-back, two children can tune into and synchronize their breaths (Goldberg 2013). Practicing breathing exercises in a group setting can promote socialization and communication. Due to their difficulties with social-relatedness, partner or group breathing activities can be particularly beneficial for children with ASD. At the age ranges discussed, verbal praise, such as "I like your smooth, soft breath," can be used to reinforce the proper execution of any of these breathing practices.

Benefits of yoga breathwork for speech sound disorders

For children with articulation and phonological issues, breathing exercises can enhance breath support for the production of sounds which require sustained airflow, such as /s/ and /z/ (Flynn 2013). Children with apraxia of speech can also benefit from breathwork. Apraxia is a speech sound disorder characterized by impairment in the precision and consistency of movements for speech in the absence of neuromuscular deficits. Children with apraxia of speech exhibit difficulty planning the spatial and temporal parameters of movement sequences, causing speech sound and prosody errors (ASHA 2007). In terms of respiration, these children can demonstrate difficulty coordinating the breath support needed to drive phonation. Repeatedly utilizing these breathing exercises could help children with apraxia of speech more accurately, consistently, and automatically produce sounds and sequences of sounds.

Summary

Yoga breathing exercises can support efficient and articulate speech production by 1) enhancing awareness of the breath, 2) strengthening and elongating trunk muscles for appropriate postural alignment, 3) improving control over the respiratory cycle, and 4) increasing the oxygen supply needed for proper functioning of the body. In addition to the benefits of breathwork related to speech sound production, these exercises which require focus on the process and products of respiration can help calm and relax children's bodies and minds, especially those with AD/HD, positively impacting language learning. The resource tables in Appendices 2–8 of this book contain information on yoga books, card decks, games, CDs, DVDs, and websites that teach many of the breathing techniques described in this chapter.

Chapter 6

YOGA FOR MOTOR PLANNING FOR SPEECH

A goal without a plan is just a wish.

attributed to Antoine de Saint-Exupéry

Introduction to motor planning

Motor planning, also called praxis, is the brain's ability to create, organize, and execute a coordinated and properly timed sequence of movements with the body (Ayres 1995). Motor planning is critical for performing daily activities such as writing, eating, brushing teeth, dressing, and tying shoes. The simple act of hand washing, for example, requires the planned execution of seven steps, namely turning on the water, obtaining soap, wetting hands, rubbing them together, rinsing hands under the water, turning off the water, and, finally, drying hands. The performance of yoga poses and speech production also require the planning of body movements in specific sequences. These motor plans must be stored in memory so that they can be retrieved when needed for future movements (O'Sullivan and Schmitz 2001). Motor planning challenges cause difficulty with initiating movements or performing them in a coordinated manner.

The production of phonetically and prosodically normal speech can be divided into four stages, namely linguistic-symbolic planning, motor planning, motor programming, and execution (Van der Merwe 2009). The first linguistic-symbolic planning stage involves all of the components of language, namely the semantic, lexical, syntactic, morphological, and phonological systems. Phonological planning involves the selection and sequencing of sounds according to the phonotactic rules of language, for example, that words in English cannot begin with the consonants "ng," "mb," or "ts."

During the motor planning stage of speech production, a plan of action reflecting motor goals is formulated (Van der Merwe 2009). The production of each speech sound involves temporal-spatial (place and manner of articulation) motor goals that are articulator rather than muscle specific. For example, the motor goals for the /m/ sound are lip closure, soft palate (velar) opening to allow airflow through the nostrils, and vocal fold closure. During this motor planning stage, the different motor goals for each speech sound are identified and the movements required for their production are sequenced. Coarticulation, which is the influence of one speech sound on another (Bauman-Waengler 2012), is also a factor during this motor planning stage. For example, the motor goals for /m/ in "moo" and /m/ in "me" differ in that the lips are more rounded for the former and more spread for the latter.

During the next stage of speech production, motor plans are converted into motor programs (Van der Merwe 2009). Motor programming for speech production involves selecting and sequencing movements for the muscles of articulation, including those of the vocal folds. This process is affected by muscle tone as well as the rate, direction, and range of movements.

Motor plans and programs are transformed into actual movements during the execution stage of speech production (Van der Merwe 2009). Although motor plans and programs are established before speech movements begin, they can be adjusted based on auditory, tactile, and proprioceptive feedback either prior to or during execution (Duffy 2012; Van der Merwe 2009). This sensory input is an important component of the motor control and coordination for speech production.

Motor planning in yoga

Yoga provides opportunities to practice the motor planning, programming, and execution of poses, breathing techniques, and chanting. As noted in Chapter 3, children's yoga classes typically include various routines, such as beginning a class with a sun salutation series of poses and concluding with a "Namaste" chant. The consistency and repetition present in a yoga practice are necessary for children to learn the motor sequences and store them in memory so that they can be retrieved for subsequent use.

The practice of individual and sequenced yoga poses presents opportunities for gross and fine motor planning and programming. Gross motor planning involves the large muscles of the torso, arms, and legs; fine motor planning uses small muscles such as those of the fingers and toes. Children must organize body movements to execute and transition both within a pose and between poses. For example, flower is an individual pose that requires several different movements. When children execute this pose, they sit down, bend their knees, place their arms underneath their legs, turn their palms face up, and balance on their buttocks, as illustrated in Figure 6.1. For the transition from mountain to chair, two different poses, children bend their knees then lift their arms, as seen in Figure 6.2.

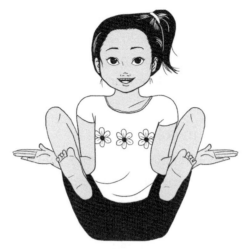

Figure 6.1 Flower pose

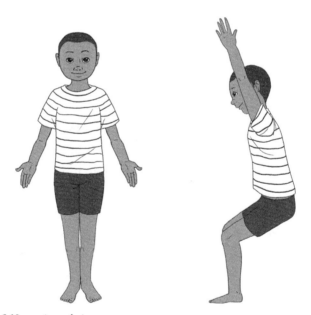

Figure 6.2 Mountain to chair pose

"Follow the Leader" imitation games improve gross motor planning skills (Goldberg 2013). In one adaptation, called "Yoga Freeze," first a leader says "go," then the children follow the leader around the room by walking, running, dancing, hopping, crawling, or moving in various ways. The movements could include "yoga walks," such as downward facing dog, lizard, or warrior I walks. When the leader shouts "freeze" and names a yoga pose, the children execute the posture.

Similar to the performance of yoga poses, the movements associated with the breathing exercises involve motor planning and programming. Children must sequence actions in order to execute various techniques. For example, as described in Chapter 5, alternate nostril breathing requires children to sequence eight steps, as shown in Box 6.1.

BOX 6.1 The eight steps of alternate nostril breathing

1. Bring the right hand in front of the face with the thumb adjacent to the right nostril and the ring finger adjacent to the left nostril.

2. Close the right nostril with the thumb.

3. Inhale through the left nostril.

4. Close the left nostril with the ring finger.

5. Exhale through the right nostril.

6. Inhale through the right nostril.

7. Close the right nostril with the thumb.

8. Exhale through the left nostril.

In order to practice "whale breath," another breathing exercise mentioned in Chapter 5, children first inhale through their nose, then tilt their head back to exhale through a "blowhole" made with cupped hands. Figure 6.3 illustrates a boy practicing whale breath.

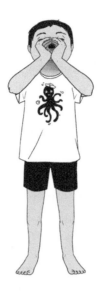

Figure 6.3 Whale breath

Motor planning for speech in yoga

Children's yoga practice can include chanting, a series of syllables or words sung either on the same note or a narrow range of notes. Chanting is not unique to yoga. In fact, it is commonly observed during sporting events and religious services. Yogic chanting provides an opportunity for children to execute motor planning and programming for speech. The neural substrates for these functions are located in the left hemisphere of the brain, especially the prefrontal, premotor cortex. Broca's area and the supplementary motor area are the most notable parts of the brain for speech production (Duffy 2012; Van der Merwe 2009). Recent research using positron emission tomography (PET) scans of individuals engaged in chanting indicated increased blood flow to the areas of the left hemisphere responsible for language processing. Moreover, repeated chanting of a mantra (sound, syllable, word, or group of words) resulted in increased blood flow to the motor cortex areas associated with movements of the mouth, including Broca's area

(Restak and Grubin 2001). Additional research is needed to define the relationship between Broca's area and developmental processes involving motor planning for speech (Love 2000).

In order to produce smooth, connected speech, the brain needs to plan the movements of the various articulators, such as the jaw, lips, and tongue. Over the course of motor speech development, children produce increasingly complex syllabic structures. Although this developmental sequence varies among children, the typical pattern of syllabic structures in order of emergence, where "C" represents "consonant" and "V" represents "vowel," is: V, CV, VC, CVC, CVCV, and CVCVC (Bleile 2004). Numerous yogic chants contain these syllabic structures and provide an opportunity to practice the sequencing of sounds.

Due to yoga's geographic roots in India, most yogic chants are written and recited in Sanskrit, an ancient, classical, literary language of the country. Table 6.1 presents some common yoga chants appropriate for children, along with their syllabic structures and meanings.

Table 6.1 Common yoga Sanskrit chants, their syllabic structure, and meanings

Sanskrit chant	Syllabic structure	Meaning
Sa ta na ma	CV	"Sa" means infinity, "ta" means life, "na" means death, and "ma" means rebirth.
Jai ma	CV	"Jai" means "victory," and "ma" means "mother."
Om	VC	"Om," also written "aum," is the universal sound.
Lam vam ram yam ham	CVC	The bija, or "seed" mantras, correspond to the chakras, or energy centers in the body.
Sat nam	CVC	"Sat" means "truth," and "nam" means "name."

cont.

Sanskrit chant	Syllabic structure	Meaning
Hari om	CVCV VC	"Hari" means "the remover," and "om" is the universal sound.
Soham	CVCVC	"Soham" means "I am He/That."
Om shanti	VC CVCCV	"Om" is the universal sound, and "shanti" means "peace."

C = consonant; V = vowel

Multisensory modalities

During learning activities, the engagement of multiple senses enhances the processing, storage, and retrieval of information. According to the principle of dual coding (Clark and Paivio 1991), information entering the nervous system through multiple processing channels helps bypass the restricted processing capacities of each individual channel. More information can be processed when disseminated between several senses. In addition, multisensory processing reduces the cognitive load, or the amount of effort used in working memory, because information from different modalities is more readily held in short-term memory and can be used to build long-term representations (Bagui 1998).

Learning and recalling the motor plans and programs for various yogic chants can be enhanced by appealing to multiple sensory processing channels, including the auditory, visual, tactile, and/or kinesthetic modalities. In order to combine modalities, children could pair their production of syllables or words by simultaneously drawing, tapping on, or moving parts of their body, or banging a gong, Tibetan "singing" bowl, or drum. For example, children could verbalize the two syllables in "shanti" while tapping their legs two times. Similarly, children could pair the verbalization of "sa ta na ma" with finger movements. During the production of the syllable "sa," the children touch their index finger to their thumb. For "ta," they touch their middle finger to their thumb. For "na," they touch their ring finger to their thumb. For "ma," they touch their pinkie finger to their thumb. These examples involve the pairing of the auditory and tactile-kinesthetic modalities, which is consistent with the notion of using multiple sensory processing channels to maximize learning.

Benefits of yoga for childhood apraxia of speech

As mentioned in Chapter 5, apraxia is a speech sound disorder involving impairment in the precision and consistency of movements for speech in the absence of neuromuscular deficits, such as abnormal tone or reflexes (ASHA 2007). Children with apraxia exhibit difficulty with motor planning and programming for speech, resulting in reduced intelligibility. The performance of yoga poses, breathing exercises, and chants presents children with apraxia the opportunity to practice and master the motor planning, programming, and execution of sequenced movement. Chanting, in particular, is beneficial for children with apraxia of speech because rhythmic treatment approaches are shown to improve functional speech production (ASHA 2007). As previously described in this chapter, multisensory cueing, such as pairing sound sequences with finger gestures, helps children with apraxia learn and retain new speech production skills. In addition, as children with apraxia benefit from repeated practice, the routines present in yoga classes offer them the opportunity to master various motor plans.

Summary

Children's yoga provides abundant opportunities to practice and master the planning, programming, and execution of gross and fine (including speech) movements. Specifically, the repetition of poses, breathing techniques, and chants present in children's yoga practice permits the brain and body to sequence movements and retain those sequences for future use. In addition, the pairing of speech with yoga movements, such as simultaneously chanting words and tapping legs or striking a "singing" bowl, increases the learning and retention of motor plans and programs by utilizing the auditory, visual, tactile, and/or kinesthetic modalities. The resource tables in Appendices 2–8 of this book contain information on yoga books, card decks, games, CDs, DVDs, and websites to enhance motor planning for speech in children.

Chapter 7

YOGA FOR VOCABULARY AND LINGUISTIC CONCEPTS

A thought unembodied in words remains a shadow.

Lev S. Vygotsky

Introduction to vocabulary development

As noted in Chapter 2, infants typically transition from the intentional prelinguistic stage to the one-word linguistic stage around the time of their first birthdays. This remarkable achievement marks the onset of vocabulary development, which continues throughout the lifespan. Children's knowledge of the words that they understand and produce is called the mental lexicon (Pence Turnbull and Justice 2017). This dictionary in the mind consists of word meanings—ideas about objects (e.g. chair), actions (e.g. bend), locations (e.g. next to), directions (e.g. up), feelings (e.g. happy), and many other notions. In the early stages of vocabulary development, children's meanings for the words they have acquired do not necessarily match the meanings the words have for adults. For example, children might use a word too broadly such as calling all furry animals "dog," or too narrowly by using the word "dog" to refer to only the family dog but not others. An important task for children in the semantic domain is the development of categorical concepts such as the knowledge that the word "chair" refers to a whole class of chairs (including lounge chairs, desk chairs, and even high chairs) and to extend the word "chair" to new, perhaps less familiar, exemplars of the object (such as beanbag chairs). Child language researchers have proposed various hypotheses about the nature of the conceptual basis of children's early word meanings, which is beyond the scope of this chapter. However, they generally agree that, in addition to meaning, children's mental lexicons contain both phonological and grammatical information including a word's part of speech (Pence Turnbull and Justice 2017). Children with a variety of neurodevelopmental challenges including language disorders, intellectual disability, autism spectrum disorder (ASD), and attention deficit/hyperactivity disorder (AD/HD) can have problems with the acquisition and use of vocabulary and its related linguistic concepts. For many of these children, first words often have a late onset, and new words are acquired more slowly than in typical development. Lexical acquisition is often targeted in language intervention for these children.

In discussing children's mental lexicons, the distinction between comprehension and production must be considered. Children's receptive vocabularies (the words they understand) often precede and exceed their expressive lexicons (the words they use). In terms of development, children typically begin to understand words before they have begun to talk, and they usually comprehend more words than they say at any point in development. However, this is not always the case. For example, some words understood are not necessarily produced, and some words that children produce are not fully understood. Bloom and Lahey (1978) suggested that these differences occur because comprehension and production represent distinct although interdependent processes in language acquisition. In addition, children with ASD might say words spontaneously or imitatively without understanding what they mean. Such imitations are considered echolalia, the repetition of another's prior utterance, which is a salient feature of some children with ASD (Kim *et al.* 2014). Immediate echolalia refers to repetitions that directly follow another's utterance (e.g. Adult: "Let's do chair pose"; Child: "Let's do chair pose"). Delayed echolalia refers to repetitions that are removed from the time and place in which they were initially heard (e.g. Child says "Sit on your mat," a phrase that the child heard on a prior occasion). Delayed echolalia sometimes originates in scripted forms of language such as movies, television commercials, or YouTube videos.

In terms of the five components of language introduced in Chapter 2, the lexicon is generally considered part of the semantic domain because, as noted above, words represent ideas or knowledge about objects, relationships, and events in the world (Bloom and Lahey 1978). However, the specific lexical items, or words, that are actually said (or signed) are considered part of morphological form (Bloom and Lahey 1978). As noted in Chapter 2, the form of words can be categorized in terms of traditional parts of speech such as nouns, pronouns, verbs, adjectives, adverbs, and prepositions. Common nouns comprise the majority of word types that children acquire first, and they continue to dominate their lexicons by the time their productive vocabularies exceed the 600-word level (Bates *et al.* 1994).

In addition to whole words, parts of words, including noun, verb, and adjective suffixes, are another type of form that children acquire. These inflectional and derivational morphemes, lexical items, and the linguistic concepts that they represent, develop in an integrative, synergistic way. Simply put, vocabulary development must be considered in relation to other language components—syntactical, morphological, phonological, and pragmatic—as well as the broader context of other developmental domains—the social-emotional, cognitive, and linguistic (Uccelli, Rowe, and Pan 2017).

Lexical growth

Following the emergence of the first few words at about one year, children's lexicons typically increase at a remarkable rate to about 300 words by age two. Throughout the toddler, preschool, and school-age years into adolescence, and even into adulthood, human beings continue to expand their vocabularies and related conceptuals. According to an estimate of lexical acquisition that focuses on the early childhood years (Biemiller 2005), children learn an average of 860 new words annually between the ages of one and seven years. According to Nippold (2007), typically developing five-year-olds know the meanings of at least 10,000 words. Further, once children have begun to read, their vocabularies increase even more rapidly with word learning occurring through the written as well as spoken modality. Nagy and Scott (2000) note that school-age children acquire about 2000 to 3000 new words each year. This translates into learning approximately five to eight new words daily!

Beyond first words

In discussing semantic development beyond the period of initial vocabulary acquisition, Uccelli *et al.* (2017) distinguish between vocabulary breadth (the number of words known) and vocabulary depth (the degree of various types of word knowledge such as multiple meanings). They note that, over time, inputs to children's vocabulary development broaden from the home environment to include other sources such as school and peer interactions. Further, vocabulary knowledge is a key factor in the development of children's literacy skills and academic success.

Yoga and vocabulary/linguistic concepts

Yoga classes for children provide an engaging source of input to support the expansion of children's vocabulary and conceptual development (Goldberg 2013; Williams 2010). The particular vocabulary words chosen by the adult who leads a class or session will vary with the children's chronological age and developmental level. Children's exposure to new words through yoga can increase the breadth of their lexical knowledge. For example, children could learn that the word "cobra," the name of a yoga pose, refers to a type of snake or that the terms "vertical" and "horizontal" refer to positions in space. In addition, they could be exposed to previously acquired, familiar words such as "chair" in new contexts and have the opportunity to embody them through the poses and breathing exercises, which increases the depth of their semantic development. Tables 7.1 to 7.3 list vocabulary words and linguistic concepts related to children's yoga practice. Although this list is not exhaustive, it provides the reader with an idea of the extent of the richness of the vocabulary and linguistic concepts that are available through children's yoga.

During a yoga class, children hear the names of the poses and the verbal directions needed to execute them, which can enhance their receptive language development. Both the names of the poses and the accompanying directions provide rich sources of vocabulary input for familiar words in new contexts (new functions for old forms) and exposure to new lexical items. The names of the yoga poses are nouns from a variety of categories including animals, elements of nature, types of furniture, transportation items, and other objects. The directions for the poses include the names of relevant body parts including hands, arms, legs, feet, toes, shoulders, neck, head, and belly. Directions for some of the breathing exercises described in Chapter 5 include the names of parts of the face (nose, mouth, and cheeks) in addition to parts of the body such as the lungs or abdomen.

Yoga poses represent several different categories of nouns. Many are named for animals such as the lion, fish, lizard, cat, cow, eagle, frog, pigeon, crocodile, and rabbit. Poses such as butterfly and locust are names of insects. Two poses, downward facing dog and upward facing dog, contain terms for directionality in addition to the animal name. Several yoga poses, such as mountain, tree, flower, and rainstorm, refer to elements of nature. Six yoga poses have the names of items of furniture: table, bench, chair, rocking chair, bed, and couch. Additional yoga poses that are practiced in children or family yoga classes are bridge, wheel, stick, bow, boat, candle, baby, and child. The names of some yoga poses that are regularly experienced in classes for children are listed in Table 7.1. In addition to these nouns, many body parts are regularly named while the yoga teacher provides the instruction for the poses. For example, when providing directions for mountain pose, the teacher can name the legs, feet, toes, shoulder, arms, hands, fingers, and head, which are all involved in practicing this pose. The names of body parts that frequently accompany teacher instructions for a variety of children's yoga poses are listed in Table 7.1.

Table 7.1 Nouns in different categories related to children's yoga practice

Body parts	Animals	Nature	Furniture	Transportation	Other objects
arm	bear	boulder	bed	airplane	bow
belly/ abdomen	butterfly	cactus	bench	bicycle	bridge
cheek	camel	flower	chair	boat	candle
chin	cat	half moon	couch	canoe	fountain
eye	cobra/ snake	lightning bolt	rocking chair	car	gate
foot	cow	log	table	chopper	phone
finger	crocodile	lotus		motorcycle	plow
hand	dog	moon		rocket ship	rag doll
head	dolphin	mountain		sailboat	slide
hip	eagle	rainbow		submarine	staff/stick
knee	elephant	rainstorm			wheel
knuckle	fish	rock			
leg	frog	seed			
mouth	giraffe	star			
neck	gorilla	sun			
nose	hare/ rabbit/ bunny	tree			
palm	lion	volcano			
shoulder	lizard				
thigh	locust				
toe	monkey				
tongue	pigeon				
wrist	stork				
	tiger				
	turtle				

The instructions for yoga poses contain many verbs. Verbs are a particularly challenging type of word for children with specific language impairment (Leonard 2014). The poses typically begin with an initial verb such as "sit," "stand," or "lie down." The directions also include other verbs, which code the actions that accompany the subsequent movements of a particular pose. In moving into yoga poses, children are often directed to bend, stretch, lift, squeeze, extend, and touch various body parts while they are reminded to breathe in and out. For school-age children, the verbs "inhale" and "exhale" could be used for the direction of the breath. For example, in an adaptation of lizard pose, children begin by lying prone on their abdomens with hands under their shoulders and fingers stretched out. The toes are bent forward; arms and legs are straight. Shoulders are drawn back and away from the ears. To add more vocabulary—and some fun— children could be instructed to stick their tongue in and out in hope of catching a bug for a snack (Wenig 2003). For school-age children, the more sophisticated verbs "protrude," "retract," and "extend," as well as the noun "insect," could be used to enhance children's lexicon during this activity. Figure 7.1 illustrates a boy in lizard pose hoping to catch a bug!

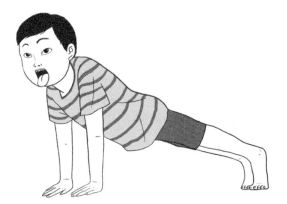

Figure 7.1 Lizard pose

For another example, in airplane pose, children first lie prone on their abdomens, then extend their arms and legs while simultaneously lifting their head. The adult could vary the sophistication of the verb (or any other word type) depending on the cognitive-linguistic development of the children's vocabulary. For example, some airplanes might "fly" whereas others might "soar." Table 7.2 lists verbs that are named as part of the directions for many children's yoga poses.

Table 7.2 Verbs related to children's yoga practice

balance	crawl	hum	release	stand	tip
bend	elevate	lean	rub	stomp	tip-toe
blow	extend	open	scan	stop	touch
breathe	flex	point	shake	stretch	twist
climb	hide	reach	shift	squeeze	walk
close	hug	relax	sit	tap	wiggle

The instructions for yoga poses and breathing exercises contain additional lexical items that code a variety of linguistic concepts. These include prepositions that code spatial/positional concepts, temporal notions, and a variety of attributes. Ristuccia (2010) discusses the use of the yoga poses to teach opposites, attributes, and other categories of words to children. In a pose specifically developed for children called "butterfly hands" (Goldberg 2013), children pretend that their hands are butterflies, flying them "in front," "in back," out to the "sides," and "all around." Similarly, a small object such as a beanbag or a toy boat, can go "under" children in bridge pose. Figure 7.2 illustrates a boy in bridge pose with a small toy boat placed underneath his body.

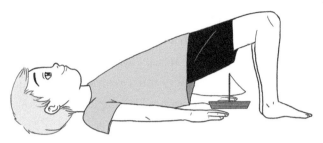

Figure 7.2 Bridge pose with toy boat

The beanbag could also be used to identify the place on someone's body where the object is balanced such as "on my shoulder" or "on his thigh" incorporating locatives, personal pronouns, and the names of body parts. School-age children could also be instructed to go "through" a tunnel created by a child (or adult) who is positioned in an inverted "L" shape, or handstand, against the wall.

Several of these words coding linguistic concepts comprise polar opposites. These antonym pairs include the spatial/positional terms "up" and "down," the temporal terms "before" and "after," and the modifiers "big" and "small." While providing the instructions for mountain pose, for example, the adult could ask the children if they are "big" or "small" mountains, using adjectives to modify the noun. While leading children into airplane pose, the modifiers "left" and "right" could be used to enhance vocabulary as the children alternate leaning in opposite directions. The temporal pairs "first" and "then" as well as "before" and "after" could be incorporated into yoga classes as the adult describes a sequence of poses, breathing exercises, or directions related to the children's movements. Table 7.3 lists the lexical items that code these additional linguistic concepts.

Table 7.3 Additional words and linguistic concepts related to children's yoga practice

Spatial	Temporal	Attributes	Colors	Shapes	Numbers
above/below	before/after	gentle	blue	circle	one
forward/backward	first/then	light/dark	green	diamond	two
in front of/behind		light/heavy	orange	triangle	three
in/on		peaceful	red		four
in/out		round	violet/purple		five
on/off		shallow/deep	white		six
right/left		short/long	yellow		seven
side		short/tall			eight
through		slow/fast			nine
together		small/big			ten
top/bottom		smooth			
under/over		soft			
up/down		strong			
vertical/horizontal		warm/cool			

Color names, another type of attribute, could also be incorporated into yoga classes. For example, children could be asked to name the color of their airplane, boat, butterfly, bridge, table, chair, flower, or other relevant pose. Further, the adult could engage the children in a practice related to the chakras, a system of seven energy centers, which, according to yoga philosophy (Simpkins and Simpkins 2011; Williams 2010), are associated with a particular color and sound. For example, the color blue and the Sanskrit consonant-vowel-consonant syllable "ham" (pronounced /ham/) are related to the fifth chakra, which is associated with the anatomical region of the throat and the act of communication. An adult might name the seven colors of the chakra system during a chant associated with this system exposing the child to the color words in a new context. This is another example of the developmental principle of old forms for new functions.

Numbers are another conceptual domain that could also be incorporated into children's yoga practice. This could be achieved in various ways. The number modifiers "first" through "seventh" could be named in conjunction with each of the chakras. In addition, the numbers one through ten could be named as children spread their fingers or toes for various poses. For example, children could count their ten fingers as they spread them for the cat-cow sequence. Similarly, children could count their ten toes as they lift and spread them for mountain pose. They could also count as they extend their ten fingers pretending to grow leaves from their branches in tree pose. Using yoga to facilitate pretend play will be the focus of the next chapter.

Numerical concepts could be incorporated as children practice rocket ship pose, which involves starting in chair pose, then bending their legs deeper and lowering their body toward the floor as they count down from ten to zero at which point they blast off by "shooting" their body toward the sky. Numerical concepts could also be integrated as children silently count the duration of the inhalation and exhalation phases of their breathing cycle while the adult guides this activity by counting out loud (Garabedian 2008). The adult could count out loud for a number of seconds while children hold a new or familiar pose (Flynn 2013). In this instance, the adult provides a model of the numbers while the child listens. A children's version of the sun salutation that has the tune of the familiar children's rhyme "one-two buckle my shoe" provides another opportunity to practice the numbers one through ten.

Shape is another conceptual-linguistic domain that could be incorporated into children's yoga practice. Triangle pose is named for the shape made by the arms and legs while in this pose. Wenig (2003) describes two seated adaptations of this pose that children practice with partners and a third standing version that is practiced individually. In downward facing dog pose, the children's straightened arms and legs form an inverted letter "V" or triangle shape. In conjunction with the opening line of a preschool level adaptation of sun salutation (Bersma and Visscher 2003), which begins "I make a circle nice and round," children form a circle with their arms. A subsequent refrain of this sun salutation states that "Now I am a triangle with my bottom on the top," which includes spatial/positional terms in addition to the name of the shape.

The comparative and superlative adjective suffixes "-er" and "-est" could be applied to many of the attributes listed in the table. For example, children can be instructed to vigorously rub their hands together "fast" and then "faster," so that when they subsequently place their opened palms over their eyes as part of a relaxation exercise, they feel "warm" or perhaps "warmer" than they did before. Similarly, children could be instructed to conduct particular actions associated with a yoga pose through songs such as Laurie Berkner's "The Airplane Song" or Karma Kids Yoga's "Tic-Toc, Little Yoga Clock" by moving faster or slower, and then the fastest or slowest. Exposure to these derivational morphemes enhances both the depth and breadth of children's lexical knowledge as they hear new words based on root words such as "fast" and "slow" from which they originated.

At the beginning or conclusion of many children's yoga sessions, a Namaste song is sung as an acknowledgement of respect to the other participants in the group. "Namaste" is a Sanskrit greeting that means "I honor the light in you" (Williams 2010). Adaptations of this salutation in children's songs include

"The light in *me* sees the light in *you*; Bow to *me*; I'll bow to *you*" (Wenig 2003). The lyrics of Kira Willey's version include the line "I honor *you* as *you* honor *me*." In yet another Namaste song, which is sung to the tune of "The Wheels on the Bus" by Karma Kids Yoga, the words state "*My* little light bows to *your* little light." One commonality across the various Namaste songs is presence of the personal pronouns "I," "me," and "you" or their possessive forms "my" and "your." From a linguistic perspective, these pronouns are considered deictic terms in that they shift reference depending on the speaker-listener roles (Pence Turnbull and Justice 2017). The pronouns "I," "me," and "my" always refer to the speaker; the terms "you" and "your" always refer to the listener. Children hearing and singing these songs experience the use of these forms in a deictically appropriate way.

Children with ASD often experience challenges in using these personal deictic pronouns. Typically, they do not make the shift from second to first person pronouns, which reflects a problem in form/use interactions. For example, the child who says "you like yoga" following the adult's query, "Do you like yoga?" uses the latter part of the prior adult utterance for his own. This atypical language behavior reflects the child's difficulties with deixis described above (Kim *et al.* 2014). In the foregoing example, the child did not make the deictic shift from person spoken to, the second person, in which the pronoun "you" is appropriate, to the speaker role, the first person, in which the pronoun "I" is correct. Linguistically, the child mistakenly uses these pronouns as if they were static forms with stable referents rather than as dynamic forms, which shift with speaker-listener discourse role. Shifting reference is particularly difficult for children with ASD because of their difficulty with abstraction and lack of flexibility (Paul and Norbury 2012). Like echolalia, these errors do not occur in all children with ASD, but are more common in individuals with autism than in other clinical populations (Kim *et al.* 2014).

Summary

Yoga practice provides a context that can enhance lexical and conceptual development in children in an engaging, enjoyable way. Yoga practice with children led by a knowledgeable, creative adult 1) exposes them to new words and 2) provides them with new functions in which previously acquired lexical items are used. These new forms and functions expand the depth and breadth of children's semantic and related conceptual knowledge. Through yoga, children are exposed to a variety of nouns, verbs, locatives, including polar opposites, attributes that code color, shape, and numbers, as well as personal pronouns. The resource tables in Appendices 2–6 of this book contain information on yoga books, card decks, games, CDs, DVDs, and websites to enhance vocabulary and linguistic concept development in children.

Chapter 8

YOGA FOR SYMBOLIC PLAY

Play is the work of childhood.

Jean Piaget

Introduction to symbolic play

Around 18 to 24 months of age, toddlers acquire the capacity to share their experiences symbolically through language, but also through other means. One of them, symbolic play, is the capacity of children to use objects and actions to stand for other objects and actions. For example, a child might lift a block into the air pretending it is an airplane or hold it to his ear as if it were a phone. Language often accompanies these symbolic play actions. For example, the child might say "plane go" in the first example and "hi daddy" in the second. The linguist Halliday (1975) coined the term "imaginative function" to describe the use of language to accompany children's early pretend play. This imaginative function reflects children's capacity to represent their world both through words and play.

The emphasis on the importance of play in relationship to children's early language development is theoretically based on the work of Piaget (1962), a biologist who became a renowned child psychologist. According to his cognitive constructivist view, play is one of several manifestations of the symbolic function, which emerges when children have developed the capacity for mental representation. He suggests that language is the most complex of the symbolic capacities. Additional examples of the symbolic function are deferred imitation, the ability to imitate absent objects or events, and drawing. Symbolic functions such as pretend play and deferred imitation require imaginal representation, the capacity to hold an image in mind without seeing it in the present moment.

Educators from different perspectives have also stressed the importance of play. For example, Parten (1932) emphasized the development of children's socialization during play using the well-known taxonomy of solitary, parallel, associative, and cooperative play. Play also provides children with an opportunity to practice learned skills, promote abstract thought, problem solve, and increase conceptual knowledge (Ellis 1973). Westby (2000) provides a speech-language perspective on the development of children's play. She developed a scale that addresses the stages of play in relation to language development in children who are presymbolic (ages 8 months through 17 months) and symbolic (ages 17 months through 5 years).

Stages of play development

The first presymbolic stage of play development maps onto the prelinguistic intentional phase of language acquisition, which lasts from about 8 months through 12 months. The hallmark of this phase, as noted in Chapter 2, is the infant's purposeful intentional two-way communication through a variety of nonlinguistic means including gaze, gesture, and vocalization. The next presymbolic stage of play from about 13 to 17 months occurs during the one-word phase of language development when infant-toddlers acquire their first words. For children who are presymbolic, the Westby Play Scale (Westby 2000) focuses on the cognitive prerequisites to language including object permanence, means-end problem solving, and object use in addition to early communication. The symbolic stage of the scale focuses on four aspects of play that develop over eight increasingly complex phases from about 17 months through five years. Table 8.1 lists these levels of symbolic play development with a description of key behaviors that characterize each stage. Beyond the five-year level, children begin to engage in games with rules (Piaget 1962), a qualitatively different type of play, which is beyond the scope of this chapter.

Table 8.1 Symbolic levels and ages of play behaviors based on the Westby Play Scale

Level	Age	Play behaviors
I	17–19 months	Children engage in autosymbolic play in which they perform single everyday actions on themselves, with life-size, realistic props such as lying on a blanket pretending to sleep.
II	19–22 months	Children's actions extend beyond the self to include others who are passive recipients of their re-enactments of everyday activities such as pretending to read a book to another.
III	24 months	Children continue to re-enact everyday activities directed toward others; they sequence two steps in play such as stirring food before pretending to feed their parent or other play partner.
IV	30 months	Children re-enact previously experienced, memorable isolated events such as getting a shot with role shifting as between doctor and patient.
V	3 years	Children combine scripts into evolving sequences such as cooking, serving, and cleaning up and assume various roles in play.
VI	3–3½ years	Children use less realistic props including miniatures and abstract representations; they re-enact events, which they may have observed but did not directly participate in. Children plan, self-monitor, and negotiate in play.
VII	3½–4 years	Children plan and improvise play themes involving multiple characters; they use dolls and replica figures to act out entire scripts; they understand characters' thoughts and feelings in addition to their actions; they hypothesize possibilities and predict outcomes.
VIII	5 years	Children re-enact novel events, which they have neither participated in nor observed. They use language rather than rely on props to plan and monitor the roles and actions of others in addition to themselves.

(adapted from Westby 2000)

Play-language relationships

Westby (2000) suggests varied relationships between language abilities and play skills in children. For most typically developing children and those with intellectual disabilities, play and language are usually at commensurate levels because of the close relationship between language and cognition. The language skills of typically developing children from verbally rich environments, however, may be more advanced than their play. Westby notes that in children with specific language impairment and speech sound disorders, play skills are usually more advanced than their linguistic form, but at similar levels to their language content and use. For verbal children with autism spectrum disorder (ASD), linguistic form is usually more advanced than play skills and at similar levels to their content and use. They may produce scripted language that is syntactically complex but said without understanding their meaning. The literature indicates that children with ASD engage in more solitary, constructive play of a repetitive nature (Kasari and Chang 2014) and less parallel, cooperative, or symbolic play of a dynamic, creative nature.

Dimensions of play

In addition to the play levels, Westby (2000) describes four dimensions of play, namely decontextualization, thematic content, organization, and self-other relations. Each of these aspects of symbolic play will be characterized and their relevance to children's yoga practice will be explained.

Decontextualization

The first dimension, decontextualization, refers to the types of props that children use to support their pretend play activities. These props, which can be identified along a continuum from realistic, to abstract, and finally invented, provide different degrees of environmental support. For example, a two-year-old child could pretend to talk on the telephone with a toy that is realistic looking and mirrors the size of the real object. The three-year-old child could use an abstract object such as a block to substitute for a telephone. At the highest level of decontextualization, the five-year-old child could pretend to talk without any prop but rather on an imaginary telephone invented in his mind. Over time, pretend play occurs with decreasing environmental support (Westby 2000), which reflects increasing decontextualization. In yoga, children primarily use their bodies in abstract ways to represent many objects including transportation items and animals, which are listed in Table 7.1 in the previous chapter on vocabulary and linguistic concepts. For example, in practicing jellyfish pose, the child lies supine on his back moving his arms and legs in a loose and floppy manner to mirror long tentacles. The adult can add language to the child's movement by encouraging him to "float and flow with no particular place to go" (Flynn 2013, p.156).

Around three years of age children become less dependent on realistic, life-size props. Instead, they can use miniature props and engage in object transformations (Westby 2000). A yoga mat and replica toys such as stuffed animals can be used as abstract representations that support yoga poses and breathing exercises. As noted in Chapter 5, a soft toy such as a rubber duck placed on the child's abdomen can be used to visualize the movement of the inhalation and exhalation phases of the breathing cycle as the toy moves up and down. As another example, small props such as a toy bird, squirrel, raccoon, or egg in a nest could be placed on the child's head to foster balance in tree pose.

In addition to defining the space for a child's practice, a yoga mat could serve as a prop that stands for various objects. It could represent a surfboard for both the standing version of surfer pose, which resembles warrior II, and for another variation of the pose in which the child lies on his stomach riding the waves. Figure 8.1 depicts two girls practicing these variations of surfer pose.

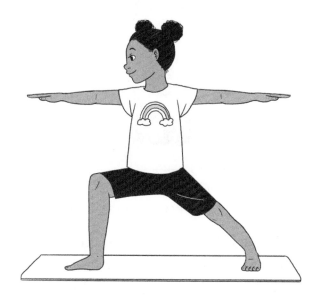

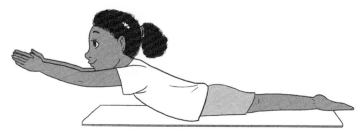

Figure 8.1 Two variations of surfer pose

A rolled-up yoga mat could represent a branch for a child squatting down in owl pose (Flynn 2013). Figure 8.2 illustrates a boy practicing this pose.

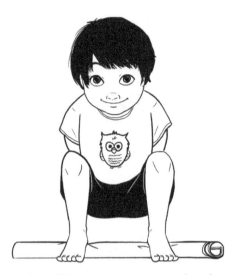

Figure 8.2 Owl pose with a rolled-up mat to represent a tree branch

The yoga mat could also serve as an abstract type of boat such as a canoe, kayak, rowboat, or sailboat as the child assumes the relevant pose. In a yoga journey activity the yoga mat could represent a magic carpet for a flying carpet ride, which transports the child to various imagined destinations. In terms of adding language, children could name and elaborate on the different sights they encounter along their journeys, which supports decontextualization and expressive language. The emergence of decontextualized language in play after three years of age is related to later success in literacy (Westby 2000). Emergent literacy skills, a precursor to reading and writing, will be addressed in the following chapter.

Miniature replicas of animals or objects can serve as props for three- to four-year-old children who could perform the pose of an animal or object selected from a small bag or other container such as a pillowcase. This can be done with a group or adult-child dyad. For example, if the child chooses a miniature toy table from the bag, the child or group of children perform a flat back table pose. To extend this activity, other children can pretend to set the table by choosing miniature-sized items for the place setting—a plastic fork, knife, spoon, and plate (Flynn 2013). Children who are already familiar with the names of the poses could guess the pose being performed by the child who chose it. In this procedure, the child who correctly names the pose chooses the next item from the bag. This activity could continue until all children have had a turn or all items have been selected. The members of an adult-child dyad could take turns practicing the pose selected from the bag.

It is well established that many children with ASD are visual learners. Picture symbols such as those available in yoga card decks can serve as visual cues. Children with intellectual disabilities would also benefit from having a concrete representation of poses, such as miniature replicas, as this population has challenges in abstract thinking. Adult models of poses can serve as a cue for all children, including those with language disorders, intellectual impairment, ASD, and attention deficit/hyperactivity disorder (AD/HD).

Thematic content

The second dimension, thematic content, refers to the schemas and scripts that are represented in play (Westby 2000). These develop from familiar, everyday activities in which the child has been an active participant (e.g. eating food) to less frequently occurring but memorable events (e.g. visiting the doctor). The thematic content of children's play can include events they have experienced, those they have observed, and eventually some which are invented. For example, when children pretend to go to the doctor, they re-enact a less frequently occurring event, but one that they would likely have previously experienced. When children pretend they are going on a space adventure, they represent an event they might have previously observed through a television program, cartoon, or movie, or read about in a book. Examples of invented themes include an imaginary safari into the jungle or a journey into the depths of the sea.

As noted in the discussion of vocabulary in the previous chapter, many yoga poses are named for animals; the thematic content of children's yoga practice reflects these creatures, some of which are listed in Table 7.1 of the previous chapter. The animals represent different categories such as those that live in the jungle, on a farm, or in the sea. In addition, biological classifications such as amphibians, birds, and insects comprise other animal categories that reflect poses in children's yoga practice. Table 8.2 lists the names of poses that belong to these different animal categories. The poses could be practiced singularly or several animals belonging to the same category could be practiced sequentially. Poses named for elements of nature, transportation, and furniture are categories that were introduced in the previous chapter. These provide additional thematic content to children's yoga practice. Children could pretend to be a basic boat or a more specific boat such as a sailboat by extending one arm straight up into the air and the other straight out in front representing sails. Another example of a general pose is fish with the more specific variants including blowfish, starfish, and jellyfish. Practiced within a session, these latter poses could constitute an undersea theme. The adult leading the activity must determine that basic level vocabulary is understood before introducing more advanced lexical items in a category.

Table 8.2 Categories of animals named in yoga poses

Jungle	Farm	Sea creatures	Amphibians and reptiles	Birds	Insects
bear	cat	blowfish	alligator	crow	bumble bee
elephant	cow	clam	anaconda	eagle	butterfly
giraffe	dog	crab	cobra/snake	flamingo	caterpillar
gorilla	duck	dolphin	crocodile	ostrich	centipede
lion	pig	fish	frog	owl	cricket
monkey	rooster	jellyfish	iguana	peacock	dragonfly
tiger		lobster	lizard	penguin	firefly
		octopus		pigeon	flea
		seal		stork	grasshopper
		shark		swan	inchworm
		snail			ladybug
		starfish			locust
		sting ray			praying mantis
		turtle			scorpion
		walrus			
		whale			

In addition to animals, items of furniture, and modes of transportation, children could pretend to be an element of nature, such as a rainstorm. This could be enacted by having children tap their fingers on different parts of their body at varying speeds and levels of intensity to create a rainstorm soundscape. A group of five-year-olds who are developmentally ready to engage in cooperative play might enjoy this practice. Alternatively, the rainstorm could be created individually or by an adult-child dyad. For some yoga poses, children could add language to the physical posture. For example, when producing volcano pose, children could say words such as "bubble" and "boom" to accompany their actions using language to support their pretend play. Flynn (2013, p.143) suggests using the environmental sound "pssssh" to mimic the sound of a geyser gushing hot water and steam for a child practicing the pose of the same name.

In children's yoga, some of the same movements of the body can serve multiple poses. For example, children, especially those under three years, could wiggle their bodies as they pretend to be objects as different as jello, a rag doll, or a jellyfish. More specifically, children could pretend to be jello by wiggling their bodies while standing or sitting. Children could portray rag dolls by wiggling their bodies as they gently sway their arms and torso side-to-side while standing. This same wiggling movement could also depict a standing variation of jellyfish, a pose previously mentioned. The use of visual supports, such as picture cues, could be helpful for children with language disorders, intellectual disabilities, ASD, and AD/HD. Some children with developmental challenges might not understand that the same movement can represent different objects, which mirrors the notion in language that words such as "fall" can have multiple meanings.

Organization

The third dimension, organization, refers to the coherence and logic of play. This component concerns the schemas and sequences of children's re-enactments (Westby 2000). Children's play develops from single action schemes (e.g. pretending to stir food in a pot) to combined sequences of actions (e.g. first stirring the food and then pretending to feed it to a doll or other play partner). At more advanced levels, children have the capacity to integrate several themes into their play, such as shopping for food, cooking it, and then serving it for dinner. Such coordinated sequences, when hierarchically organized, reflect the greater complexity of symbolic play during the later preschool years. In yoga, children can move from one pose to another, creating dynamic sequences. The transition from mountain to chair is an example that was mentioned in Chapter 6 on motor planning. Another example includes the transition from candle to candelabra. Figure 8.3 illustrates a girl in candle and candelabra poses.

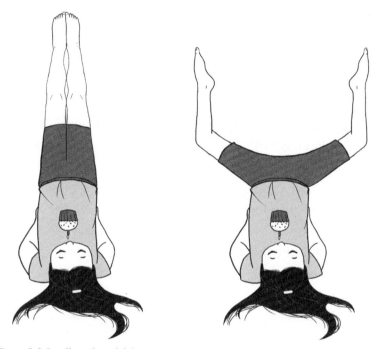

Figure 8.3 Candle and candelabra poses

The so-called "warrior" poses, commonly practiced in adult yoga, provide another opportunity for children to engage in a sequence of poses, honing the organization of their play. For these standing poses, the children begin in warrior I, move into warrior II, and if able to balance on one foot, practice warrior III. In some classes, children produce affirmations such as "I am strong! I am bold! My own balance I can hold!" to accompany this warrior sequence. Another sequence that improves organization is the sun salutation, a series of poses that is common in adult yoga practice, but can be adapted for children. Michael Chissick's *Seahorse's Magical Sun Sequences* is a delightful children's book about adapting this series of poses for children of varied abilities. Hardy (2015) presents a simplified sun salutation sequence that she uses with children with ASD and other special needs. Children with AD/HD may have difficulties sustaining attention to multistep sequential play. Engaging in yoga activities that involve multiple steps could help children from this population improve the organization of their play.

Self-other

The fourth and final dimension, self-other relations, refers to the roles that can be assumed in play interactions (Westby 2000). According to Piaget (1962), the understanding that one can assume different roles requires decentration, the capacity to understand that people sometimes have different perspectives. This aspect of play requires that children recognize the mental states of others, a social-cognitive capacity called "theory of mind" (ToM) (Premack and Woodruff 1978). Most children with ASD demonstrate challenges with ToM (Baron-Cohen *et al.* 2005; Bauminger-Zviely 2014). Consequently, they are unlikely to attribute feelings and desires to their play partners, whether dolls, toy animals, or people (Westby 2000). Yoga could provide a safe context for children with ASD to develop in ToM. Flynn (2013) describes several partner poses such as lizard on a rock, park bench, puppy friends, and see-saw that encourage teamwork and connection. These poses involve elements of reciprocity and turn-taking, aspects of social interaction and social communication discussed in Chapter 4. In addition to the communication benefits of these activities, they also enhance the self-other dimension of play.

The developmental roots of ToM emerge in the presymbolic intentional period when infants can share their attention with another regarding an object or event. This capacity for joint attention was introduced in Chapter 2. During the preschool years, children understand that they and others can have different likes, beliefs, and feelings. Recognizing these differences underlies children's ability to assume different roles in play. For example, in a patient-doctor scenario, a child could assume the role of the doctor and an adult could pretend to be the patient.

In some yoga poses, children can take on the roles of other persons. Examples of these so-called "people poses" include woodchopper, ice skater, skier, rock star, hero, archer, ninja, dancer, and baby in addition to the warriors previously mentioned in the earlier discussion of thematic content. Figure 8.4 illustrates a boy in dancer pose, one of several people poses.

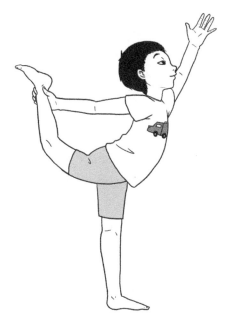

Figure 8.4 Dancer pose

The self-other dimension of play is also relevant to children's assuming the roles of both follower and leader during yoga practice. In a group context, different children could take turns leading the group. This could benefit the self-esteem of all children and provide them with a topic of conversation to share with family and friends. Within an adult-child dyad, the members could simply switch roles. Children could also take turns assigning different animal roles to other students as they act out life in the jungle, on the farm, under the sea, or in another environment. Another activity that relates to the self-other dimension of play is yoga sculpture (Yaffa and Yaffa n.d.). In this activity, one child rests in child pose while the other plays the role of the sculptor-artist, who moves the resting child, one part at a time, into a yoga pose statue. The particular pose could be derived from a card in a deck of yoga poses that the child is given or selects. Several examples of card decks of yoga poses are listed in Appendix 4 at the end of this book. The skillful adult who leads the activity needs to determine if it is developmentally appropriate, as the children would need to be familiar with the concepts of sculpture and artists.

Another idea for the facilitation of the self-other dimension of play involves two groups of children, one group that assumes the role of trees and another that pretends to be bees (Yaffa and Yaffa n.d.). This could also be accomplished with an adult-child dyad. The children who role-play the trees practice tree pose. The children who pretend to be bees move around the various trees producing a buzzing or humming sound (described as "bee breath" in Chapter 5), but do not touch them. After a few minutes, the children (or members of the adult-child dyad) switch roles. In a variation of this yoga activity, the children could enact the role of flowers while seated in flower pose.

As noted in the foregoing chapters, songs can be incorporated into children's yoga practice. For example, the familiar song "I'm a Little Teapot" can be used to enhance self-other relations in a group or dyad. Some children can pretend to be teapots and assume teapot pose. The others, who assume the role of teacups, receive imaginary tea from the teapots. Figure 8.5 depicts two girls in these poses. The children can then reverse roles so that the relatively passive teacups get to be the more active teapots. These role reversal partner yoga activities support the development of reciprocity in addition to the self-other dimension of play.

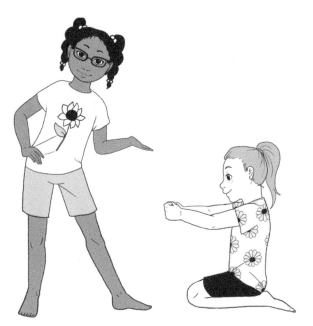

Figure 8.5 Teapot and teacup poses

Summary

Yoga provides a context for children to practice their symbolic play skills. These develop from the end of the first year of infancy through the toddler-preschool years. Based on the levels of increasing complexity delineated by Westby (2000) and theoretically grounded in a Piagetian framework (Piaget 1962), symbolic play can be characterized along the four aspects of decontextualization, thematic content, organization, and self-other. Yoga can help children who are typically developing, as well as those who are developmentally challenged, to hone their play skills in each of these four dimensions. The resource tables in Appendices 2–8 of this book contain information on yoga books, card decks, games, CDs, DVDs, and websites to enhance symbolic play development in children.

Chapter 9

YOGA FOR EMERGENT LITERACY

You're never too old, too wacky, too wild,
to pick up a book and read to a child.

Anita Merina

Introduction to emergent literacy

According to the United Nations Educational, Scientific and Cultural Organization (2004, p.13), literacy is "the ability to identify, understand, interpret, create, communicate, and compute using printed and written materials associated with varying contexts." Simply put, literacy is the ability to read and write. Children transition from emergent literacy of the preschool period to decoding the written word during the school-age years. In addition to decoding, children eventually learn to read for meaning (Justice and Pence 2005). In this chapter, we focus on the use of yoga to enhance emergent literacy, the earliest period of children's learning about written language (Pence Turnbull and Justice 2017).

From birth until kindergarten, during the emergent literacy period, children acquire certain knowledge, skills, and attitudes that are the developmental precursors to reading and writing (Whitehurst and Lonigan 1998). Developments in two interrelated areas, literacy socialization and literacy awareness (an aspect of metalinguistic awareness), begin during this period (van Kleeck and Schuele 1987). Literacy socialization refers to the cultural and social aspects of reading that children acquire by being members of a literate society. Literacy awareness refers to the knowledge of the linguistic code that children must master to become literate. These interrelated aspects of development, as shown in Figure 9.1, will be addressed in the following sections of this chapter.

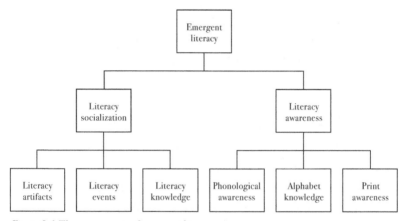

Figure 9.1 The components of emergent literacy

Literacy socialization

The first area, literacy socialization, includes three elements—artifacts, events, and knowledge, which are obtained prior to learning to read. Each of these will be described below.

Literacy artifacts

Literacy artifacts refer to representations of print that enrich children's environments (van Kleeck and Schuele 1987). Examples include pictures of characters such as Thomas the Tank Engine and logos that adorn children's bedrooms, clothes, books, toys, and food packages. Logos, a particularly important type of literacy artifact, expose children to the importance of print.

Literacy events

Literacy events, situations in which people engage with reading or writing (Heath and Street 2008), enhance and expand children's world knowledge of concepts as varied as cultural diversity, money, nature, and life issues such as birth and death. As children's worlds are often limited to their immediate environments of home, school, and community, storybooks introduce them to the broader world in which they live. For example, for children living in a land-locked area such as the central part of the United States, storybooks can teach them about coastal regions that include beaches, boats, and buoys.

Shared book reading is an established, well-researched literacy event that allows adults to create meaningful, motivating contexts for children to learn such skills (Justice and Pence 2005). Adult scaffolding of these interactions helps children attain increasingly independent, higher levels of emergent literacy. Justice and Pence (2005) identified four different types of scaffolds that adults provide during the literacy event of shared book reading: distancing, linguistic, regulatory, and structural. Distancing scaffolds involve comments on children's immediate (e.g. "I like the way you did that!") and prior past (e.g. "Remember, you've done this before") performances. Linguistic scaffolds provide more advanced models of language and literacy that build upon children's current level of knowledge or skill. Examples include asking open-ended questions (e.g. "What do you think this book is about?"), describing unfamiliar concepts (e.g. "The elephant is very big. It's gigantic!"), and extending children's talk (e.g. Child: "It's the letter T"; Adult: "It's an uppercase T"). Regulatory scaffolds help children learn how one task applies to another.

Examples include discussing how small tasks apply to larger ones (e.g. "Knowing these letters will help you read these words"), describing task components (e.g. "To read this word, you need to look at each letter"), and aiding children in reflective self-evaluation (e.g. "How do you think you did?"). Structural scaffolds refer to aspects of the context in which learning takes place that help to facilitate children's learning. Examples include working in familiar environments, incorporating motivating materials, and involving peers in shared book reading.

The literacy event of shared book reading also promotes the development of children's ability to produce their own stories, a topic that was introduced in Chapter 2 with the discussion of the emergence of narratives during the "Later Syntactic-Semantic Complexity" stage of language development (Gerber and Prizant 2000). Children's narratives, whether spoken or written, convey real or fictional events about the past, present, or future. In order to produce narratives, children must incorporate knowledge across the different domains of language—morphology, syntax, semantics, phonology, and pragmatics (Justice and Pence 2005). The written narratives contained in early chapter books often include more explicit, detailed, literate language than that found in books with an abundance of pictures, which provide a different source of context. Examples of literate, decontextualized language include elaborated noun phrases (e.g. "our new boat"), adverbial phrases (e.g. "after the sunset"), conjunctions (e.g. "although"), and specific vocabulary (e.g. "stern" and "rudder"). Adults can facilitate narrative development and literate language by exposing children to books with stories that contain temporal and causal sequences (Justice and Pence 2005).

Literacy knowledge

The third and final element of literacy socialization, literacy knowledge, refers to information that children acquire from literacy experiences with artifacts (van Kleeck and Schuele 1987) including print awareness (an aspect of literacy awareness to be discussed below) and some basic book reading conventions (Justice and Pence 2005). For example, children learn about book orientation, which includes identifying the cover and back of a book, holding it upright, and turning the pages from left to right. In English, children learn that reading occurs from top to bottom and from left to right. However, children reading Arabic, Urdu, and Hebrew, for example, learn to read from right to left. Sound-letter correspondence, the knowledge of which graphemes (letters) represent phonemes (sounds) in words, is another type of literacy knowledge that can occur within the context of literacy socialization events. Finally, literacy experiences with artifacts also teach children about the traditional parts of speech, namely nouns, pronouns, verbs, adjectives, adverbs, conjunctions, prepositions, and interjections (Justice and Pence 2005).

Literacy awareness

In addition to the different elements of literacy socialization presented in the foregoing discussion, the emergent literacy period coincides with the development of metalinguistic awareness, sometimes simply called language awareness. Language awareness for literacy involves a developing understanding of the written word. Literacy awareness is nurtured in the context of the literacy socialization events described in the previous section. Metalinguistic awareness, the understanding of language as an object in itself as a cognitive construct, rather than as a tool for communication, plays an important role in emergent literacy and later reading success (Giess 2014). Metalinguistic awareness for literacy includes phonological awareness, alphabet knowledge, and print awareness (Pence Turnbull and Justice 2017). Literacy awareness is nurtured in the context of the literacy events previously mentioned. Each of these three aspects of literacy awareness shall be discussed below.

Phonological awareness

Literacy events with artifacts, two of the three areas of literacy socialization discussed above, provide a context for the development of phonological awareness, the first aspect of metalinguistic awareness. Phonological awareness is a type of metalinguistic skill because it requires children to reflect on one aspect of language—the sound system—as an object in itself. This awareness of the sounds of spoken language is crucial for learning to read (Justice and Pence 2005).

Beginning around two years of age and continuing through the early school years, children gain sensitivity to the sound structure of words and syllables (Pullen and Justice 2003). Literacy experiences allow children to progress from an awareness of larger units of sound, such as whole words and syllables, to an awareness of smaller units, such as phonemes. Children with phonological awareness understand, for example, that "man" and "pan" are units of language called words, that words are built from units of sound, and that these words differ in one letter but share two others (Whitehurst and Lonigan 1998). Such awareness of phonemes is critical for learning to read; conversely, learning to read increases one's phoneme awareness. Table 9.1 lists some phonological awareness skills in developmental order with examples of adult procedures that can be used to elicit them.

Table 9.1 Phonological awareness skills with
examples of adult elicitation procedures

Phonological awareness skill	Adult elicitation procedures
Recognition of rhyming words	"Do 'dog' and 'shirt' rhyme?"
Production of new rhyming words	"What rhymes with 'boat'?"
Segmentation of words in sentences	"Clap for each word you hear in the sentence 'The apple is good'."
Blending of syllables	"I am going to say parts of a word. Tell me what the word is. 'Ham-ster'."
Segmentation of syllables	"Clap for each syllable you hear in the word 'kangaroo'."
Identification of words with the same beginning sound (alliteration)	"Do these words begin with the same sound or with different sounds? Wonderful Wally Walrus."
Deletion of syllables	"Say the word 'goodnight.' Now say it without saying 'good'."
Identification of sounds in words	"What sound do you hear at the end of 'music'?"
Blending of sounds	"Put these sounds together to make a word. 'C-u-p'."
Segmentation of sounds	"Tell me each sound you hear in the word 'sun'."
Deletion of sounds	"Say 'chair'. Now say it without the 'ch'."
Addition of sounds	"Say 'sun'. Now say it with an 'e' at the end."
Manipulation of sounds	"Change the 's' in 'sand' to 'l' and say the new word."

Alphabet knowledge

The second aspect of metalinguistic awareness, alphabet knowledge, includes information about the letters of the alphabet that comprises the written code. Literacy events with artifacts provide the opportunity for children to gain knowledge about the names and features of the letters of the alphabet (Giess 2014).

This knowledge includes the notion that letters or combinations of letters of the alphabet represent specific sounds and that some sounds are consonants, whereas others are vowels. When children transition from learning to read to reading to learn, more advanced levels of alphabet knowledge are required (Whitehurst and Lonigan 1998).

Alphabet knowledge is the single best predictor of elementary-grade achievement in word recognition (Adams 1990). In the early school-age years, children learn about the relationship between letters or combinations of letters (graphemes) and sounds (phonemes). Learning this alphabetic principle (Pence Turnbull and Justice 2017) is the beginning of true reading.

Print awareness

The third aspect of metalinguistic awareness, written language awareness, refers to children's knowledge of the purpose and organization of print (Justice and Pence 2005). Given adequate exposure to the written word, children learn during the emergent literacy period that print deserves special attention. They begin to understand that print gives meaning to events and details beyond other types of visual information, such as pictures. Children's knowledge of the names of the letters, words, and other print units increases throughout language literacy development. Eventually, children learn the characteristic ways in which print is organized for different types of writing (Justice and Pence 2005), such as shopping lists, and eventually for different genres, such as fiction and nonfiction.

Strategies for shared book reading

As mentioned earlier in this chapter, shared book reading is a powerful literacy event for facilitating emergent reading and writing skills. Adults can structure reading interactions with children in order to maximize benefits from this activity. Adults' sensitivity and responsivity to children during shared book reading is crucial (Justice and Pence 2005). In order to engage children, adults can sit face-to-face with them, observe their interests and actions, and listen and respond to their questions and comments. According to van Kleeck and Schuele (1987), adults can use a developmental progression of question types and comments to enhance children's language during shared book reading. Table 9.2 presents different types of adult linguistic input and the associated child language behaviors that could be elicited.

Table 9.2 Developmental progression of question types and comments that adults can use to elicit language behaviors in children during shared book reading

Children's language behaviors	Types of questions and comments
In order for children to...	*Adults could...*
label items	ask "what" or "who" questions
elaborate on items	ask specific questions regarding the number and type of items
code events	ask "What happened?"
elaborate on events	ask about locations or consequences
talk about motives or causes	ask "why" or "how" questions
react to the story	ask how the children feel about the characters and their actions
relate the story to the real world	comment on the relevance of the characters or events in the story to the real world

(adapted from van Kleeck and Schuele 1987)

It is generally helpful for adults to ask open-ended questions (e.g. "What do you see?") in order to elicit more language from children rather than yes-no questions (e.g. "Do you see a baby?"), which only require a one-word "yes" or "no" response. When asking children questions, waiting expectantly for at least ten seconds before modeling or prompting the answers is suggested. Prompting can include pointing to a word or picture, providing the first sound of the answer (e.g. Adult: "What sound does a lion make? Rrrr…"), or giving semantic clues (e.g. Adult: "What does a monkey eat? It's yellow and long"). In addition to answering questions posed by adults, it is important that children be given the opportunity to ask questions. In this way, children will have the opportunity to initiate language during shared book reading rather than just respond. Children with autism spectrum disorder (ASD) more frequently respond to language than initiate language. Opportunities for them to initiate language during literacy activities can be very beneficial.

Expansion and extension are two other language-facilitating techniques that can be used during shared book reading. Expansions are adult-contingent verbal responses that repeat a child's prior utterance while adding relevant grammatical details. Expansion involves restating and completing the child's immature utterance. For example, when the child says, "Cow eat," the adult expands the child's shorter, ungrammatical utterance to the grammatically complete "The cow is eating." Extensions, a related language-facilitating strategy, are contingent verbal responses that add semantic information to the child's prior utterance. For example, when the child says, "Cow eat," in reference to a picture in a book, the adult can add new content, such as the type of food the cow is eating as is done in the response, "The cow is eating grass." This latter example includes both grammatical expansion and semantic extension. In shared book reading contexts, adults are likely to use both of these techniques together. The embedding of expansions and extensions during shared book reading helps build competence in all language domains, including word and sentence structure, vocabulary, and pragmatics, especially back-and-forth reciprocity and topic maintenance in conversation. These language-facilitating techniques broaden the scope of children's questions and answers, which enhances overall language learning (Ristuccia 2010). The provision of specific literacy skill-related feedback is beneficial too. For example, instead of exclaiming "Great job!" the adult could say "I love the way you turn the pages in the book!" which is related to the particular literacy event at hand.

Yoga and emergent literacy

A yoga practice presents a perfect opportunity to teach children emergent literacy skills. Books can easily be incorporated into yoga sessions. Lederer (2012) suggests that books with animals or nature themes containing short, predictable lines work well. Table 9.3 lists general books that can be used to incorporate stories into children's yoga practice.

Table 9.3 Titles and authors of general books for young children that can be incorporated into a yoga practice

Title	Author
Hug	Alborough, Jez
Dear Zoo	Campbell, Rod
From Head to Toe	Carle, Eric
The Very Busy Spider	Carle, Eric
The Very Hungry Caterpillar	Carle, Eric
Calico Cat at the Zoo	Charles, Donald
All the Awake Animals Are Almost Asleep	Dragonwagon, Crescent
The Foot Book	Dr. Seuss
They Call Me Woolly: What Animal Names Can Tell Us	DuQuette, Keith
Count!	Fleming, Denise
Beast Feast	Florian, Douglas

A to Z, Do You Ever Feel Like Me? A Guessing Alphabet of Feelings, Words, and Other Cool Stuff	Hausman, Bonnie
Fish Is Fish	Lionni, Leo
Chicka Chicka Boom Boom	Martin Jr., Bill and Archambault, John
Brown Bear, Brown Bear, What Do You See?	Martin Jr., Bill and Carle, Eric
Panda Bear, Panda Bear, What Do You See?	Martin Jr., Bill and Carle, Eric
Polar Bear, Polar Bear, What Do You Hear?	Martin Jr., Bill and Carle, Eric
Jiggle, Wiggle, Prance	Noll, Sally
Baby Beluga	Raffi
Where Do Bears Sleep?	Shook Hazen, Barbara
Over in the Meadow	Wadsworth, Olive A. and Keats, Ezra Jack
I Went Walking	Williams, Sue

In addition to general children's books, a variety of yoga-specific books are widely available. These can be incorporated into children's yoga sessions for a shared book reading event. Table 9.4 lists the titles and authors of some yoga-specific books that could be used in this context.

Table 9.4 Titles and authors of yoga books for young children that can be used during shared book reading

Title	Author
My Daddy Is a Pretzel: Yoga for Parents and Kids	Baptiste, Baron
Frog's Breathtaking Speech	Chissick, Michael
Ladybird's Remarkable Relaxation	Chissick, Michael
Seahorse's Magical Sun Sequences	Chissick, Michael
Babar's Yoga for Elephants	de Brunhoff, Laurent

cont.

Title	Author
Good Night Yoga: A Pose-by-Pose Bedtime Story	Gates, Mariam
Fly Like a Butterfly	Khalsa, Shakta Kaur
Peaceful Piggy Meditation	MacLean, Kerry Lee
Kids Yoga: Bedtime Rhymes	Maier, Jeff
Dogi the Yogi	Notarile Scrivan, Maria
The ABCs of Yoga for Kids	Power, Teresa Anne
Learn with Yoga ABC Virtues	Ristuccia, Christine
Good Night, Animal World: A Kids Yoga Bedtime Story	Shardlow, Giselle
Hello, Bali: A Kids Yoga Island Adventure Book	Shardlow, Giselle
Storytime Yoga: Teaching Yoga to Children Through Story	Solis, Sydney
Little Yoga: A Toddler's First Book of Yoga	Whitford, Rebecca
You Are a Lion! and Other Fun Yoga Poses	Yoo, Tae-Eun

Books can be incorporated into the practice of yoga poses, breathing exercises, and meditation (Lederer 2012; Ristuccia 2010; Solis 2006). While reading books, adults can pause for yogic opportunities. For example, when reading *Chicka Chicka Boom Boom* by Bill Martin Jr. and John Archambault, children can practice tree pose. *I Went Walking* by Sue Williams provides a context for several different poses, namely cat, horse, cow, duck, pig, and dog. Adults can read the popular children's book *Baby Beluga* by Raffi and perform whale's breath, which was mentioned in Chapters 5 and 6. While reading *Ladybird's Remarkable Relaxation* by Michael Chissick or *Peaceful Piggy Meditation* by Kerry Lee MacLean, children can practice relaxation and meditation. Speech-language pathologist Angela Moorad's website OMazing Kids, LLC, which is listed in the web-based resource table in Appendix 8 at the end of this book, contains comprehensive wellness activities, including an extensive list of books suitable for yoga with children.

Children often desire to read books numerous times. Multiple readings of the same book allow children to gain familiarity with the vocabulary and concepts in the story while gaining confidence in their emergent literacy skills (Justice and Pence 2005). As noted in Chapter 3, children learn new skills through repetition, which is beneficial for all children including those with neurodevelopmental disabilities. Yoga classes for young children frequently involve routines, such as consistently beginning with an adapted sun salutation or concluding with a farewell song, such as "Namaste." Children with ASD, in particular, thrive in the context of routines. In yoga classes, the adult can read the same book multiple times to children who will benefit from repeated exposure to the vocabulary and concepts presented in the story. While reading the story, the adult can pause in specific places so that the children can fill in familiar words or phrases, providing them with the opportunity to express the particular lexical items they previously learned. This opportunity to practice a word or phrase is especially beneficial to children with expressive language disorders. Both typically developing children and those with neurodevelopmental disabilities can participate in literacy events in other ways, such as by opening the book and turning the pages.

As mentioned in Chapter 3, flexibility is an important characteristic of children's yoga classes. One way to be flexible is to allow children to make choices when possible. In terms of emergent literacy, children can choose between two (or more) books they would like to read. Children can also choose which pose(s) or breathing exercise(s) to practice. For example, when reading *Over in the Meadow* by Olive A. Wadsworth and Ezra Jack Keats, children can choose between practicing lizard, fish, or frog pose.

Another way to be flexible is to substitute the children's names for the characters in the story. Doing so will make the yoga-literacy experience more personal and memorable, thereby helping to maintain the children's attention (Vukelich, Christie, and Enz 2002). For example when reading *Frog's Breathtaking Speech* by Michael Chissick, a child's name could be substituted for the character "Frog." Another attention-getting technique is the use of props such as puppets that represent different characters (Flynn 2013). Incorporating them into the yoga-literacy activity helps the story come alive thereby maintaining the children's focus. For example, butterfly and caterpillar puppets can accompany the reading of *The Very Hungry Caterpillar* by Eric Carle and the practice of the corresponding poses. Figure 9.2 illustrates a girl in butterfly and caterpillar poses.

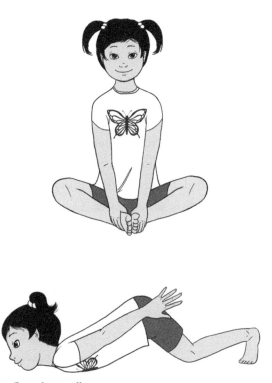

Figure 9.2 Butterfly and caterpillar poses

As discussed earlier in this chapter, phonological awareness refers to knowledge about the sound structure of language. Yoga classes provide numerous opportunities for children to develop their phonological awareness skills, especially rhyming. Children's yoga classes can include modified sun salutations paired with rhyming poems. Bersma and Visscher's (2003) *Yoga Games for Children* contains a delightfully rhyming "Salutation to the Sun."

The children's yoga book titled *ABC Virtues* by Christine Ristuccia contains rhyming poems for each letter of the alphabet that has a corresponding yoga pose or breathing exercise. Ristuccia (2010) also suggests that after children practice a yoga pose, the adult could ask them for word(s) that rhyme with the name of the pose. For example, after children practice cat pose, the adult asks, "What rhymes with *cat*?" Many popular children's songs also contain rhyming words that can be paired with yoga poses. For example, the song "I'm a Little Teapot" contains strong rhyme in the final words of each line—"stout," "spout," "shout," and "out." Figure 8.5 in Chapter 8 on symbolic play illustrates two children practicing teapot and teacup poses. Children can create yoga rhyming words, including both real words (e.g. "*Cat* on the *mat*") and non-words (e.g. "*Yoga* rhymes with *boga*, *loga*, and *moga*"). In addition to rhyming, another phonological awareness skill, syllable segmentation, can be incorporated into children's yoga practice. For example, children can tap or clap out syllables in words, such as in the yoga salutation "na-ma-ste."

Yoga classes also present the opportunity for children to gain alphabet knowledge, an important predictive emergent literacy skill described earlier in this chapter. The adult can instruct children to think of a yoga pose that begins with a letter of the alphabet. For example, if the adult says "A," the children might suggest airplane or archer poses. Yoga alphabet cards, such as Christine Ristuccia's *ABC Yoga Cards for Kids* and Teresa Anne

Power's *The ABCs of Yoga for Kids*, can also guide the children. Appendix 4 at the end of this book contains additional examples.

Another activity that can be used to foster alphabet knowledge is having the children make letters with their bodies. For example, a child practicing boat pose with raised arms forms the letter "V" with his body. Children can also practice as pairs to form letters of the alphabet. Figure 9.3 presents two boys in a partner boat pose variation to form the letter "W." Similarly, two children practicing downward facing dog pose side-by-side form the letter "M."

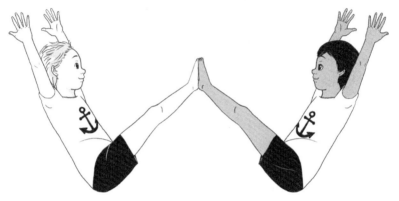

Figure 9.3 Partner boat pose variation to form the letter "W"

Yoga and emergent literacy for special populations

The yoga-literacy activities and strategies described in this chapter can benefit children who are typically developing as well as those with a variety of neurodevelopmental disabilities. Children with primary language disorders exhibit difficulty with the comprehension and production of written as well as spoken language (Paul and Norbury 2012). Children with persistent speech sound disorders, including articulatory, phonological, and praxis-based issues, are at risk for literacy problems. Children with intellectual disabilities demonstrate difficulty with academic learning, including literacy. Some children with autism spectrum disorder (ASD) show a deep interest in letters and decode words well; however, their reading comprehension skills are usually poor (Kim *et al.* 2014; Paul and Norbury 2012). In addition, they have challenges understanding the motivations and feelings of characters in narratives. Children with ASD can benefit in particular from assuming different roles during yoga-literacy activities, such as those in the character-rich fables in Solis' (2006) *Storytime Yoga™: Teaching Yoga to Children Through Story*, in order to better comprehend other people's perspectives. Rates of reading disorders are extremely high in children with attention deficit/ hyperactivity disorder (AD/HD) (Willcutt and Pennington 2000). Due to their difficulties controlling attention and behavior, children with AD/HD can present with learning problems in all academic areas, including literacy. As mentioned in Chapter 6, multisensory cueing reduces the cognitive load and actually allows more information to be processed (Bagui 1998). During yoga-literacy activities, multiple sensory processing channels (e.g. auditory, visual, tactile, and kinesthetic modalities) can be engaged by the use of music, gestures, pictures, tapping body parts, moving in poses, and breathing exercises. These supports assist children with various neurodevelopmental disabilities to build emergent literacy skills.

Summary

Emergent literacy refers to the reading and writing knowledge and skills that precede and lay the foundation for conventional literacy (Teale and Sulzby 1986). Two domains, namely literacy socialization and metalinguistic awareness, characterize the emergent literacy period. Literacy socialization describes the cultural and social aspects of reading that children learn by being a member of a literate society, whereas metalinguistic awareness includes knowledge of the linguistic code that children must master in order to become literate (van Kleeck and Schuele 1987). The practice of yoga is well suited to support both literacy socialization and metalinguistic awareness. Yoga classes are language-rich contexts, which can enhance both oral and written language development. Books can easily be incorporated into yoga classes, which can increase phonological awareness, alphabet knowledge, and print awareness. Adults can pair the practice of yoga poses, breathing exercises, and meditation with the written word in order to create experientially rich yoga-literacy activities that challenge and propel children on their journey to becoming literate members of society. The resource tables in Appendices 2–8 of this book contain information on yoga books, card decks, games, CDs, DVDs, and websites to enhance emergent literacy development in children.

SUMMARY AND CONCLUSION

In this book, we have attempted to demonstrate that the ancient tradition of yoga, which is the union of the mind, body, and spirit, is a powerful tool that can be used to enhance speech, language, and communication development in children. We have suggested that because of its flexibility in formats, including types of sessions, yoga can meet the needs of different children across the ages from birth to about twelve years of age (and beyond)—both typically developing children and those with neurodevelopmental challenges. Among the special populations that we have discussed are children with speech sound disorders, language disorders, intellectual disability, autism spectrum disorders, and attention deficit/hyperactivity disorder (AD/HD).

Amidst its growing popularity over the past twenty years, educators and clinicians in various allied professions have reported that yoga calms and organizes children's bodies and minds for effective learning, targets multiple pathways, and aids in the retention of new skills. However, as we have stressed, the contributions of yoga have rarely been examined from a speech-language perspective. As speech-language clinicians and yoga practitioner-teachers, we have repeatedly observed that yoga sessions are language-rich contexts. We have identified six areas of development related to speech, language, and communication, which we firmly believe yoga can facilitate—namely prelinguistic communication, breath support, motor planning, vocabulary/ concepts, symbolic play, and emergent literacy. With the logical relationship of yoga to these six developmental domains addressed in the foregoing chapters, and our awareness of the lack of data to support these connections in the contemporary literature, we conclude this book with a call for evidence from research-oriented children's yoga instructors and clinicians with interest in using yoga to enhance speech-language development in children. We realize that the first generation of research in this area will necessarily be exploratory, but that is an appropriate way to begin to address this potentially powerful complement to typical speech, language, and communication development as well as traditional speech-language intervention. Amidst its growing popularity, the stakeholders in this endeavor include children of all ages as well as the families and professionals who serve them. As Bill Gates (2000) noted in a keynote address, "any tool that enhances communication has profound effects in terms of how people can learn from each other, and how they can achieve the kind of freedoms that they're interested in."

PART III

APPENDICES OF YOGA RESOURCES

Appendix 1

Definitions and Examples of Developmental Domains

Communication

Communication refers to the process of sharing information among individuals. This includes both infants' intentional engagement with another through the nonlinguistic means of gaze, gestures, and vocalizations as would occur in a "Mommy and Me" yoga class, as well as verbal children's pragmatic use of language to interact with others as would occur during a partner yoga pose.

Breath support

Breath support for speech refers to the stabilization of the body for proper airflow for speech. Yoga poses can enhance breath support by strengthening and elongating the trunk muscles needed for appropriate postural alignment for efficient speech production. Breath control for speech, a related area, refers to the regulation and coordination of airflow for speech. Yoga breathing exercises can enhance breath control by increasing awareness of the breath and teaching control over the entire respiratory cycle.

Motor planning

Motor planning for speech refers to the brain's ability to create, organize, and execute coordinated and properly timed sequences of articulator (e.g. jaw, lips, and tongue) movements to produce smooth, connected speech. The repetition of yoga chants, such as "Namaste," as well as the production of words while performing yoga poses (e.g. "meow" in cat pose), provide opportunities to practice and master sequenced speech movements.

Vocabulary/concepts

Vocabulary refers to the words and concepts refer to the knowledge that underlies the words that children both understand and produce. These lexical items that children are exposed to through yoga reflect many different notions including inanimate objects such as "bridge," living creatures such as "caterpillar," actions such as "stretch," and attributions including colors and shapes, locations, directions, and feelings.

Symbolic play

Symbolic play refers to the capacity of children to use objects and actions to stand for other objects and actions. This is commonly called pretend play during the preschool years and requires the ability to hold an image in mind without seeing it in the present moment. The term imagination is often used for this same capacity at later developmental levels. Yoga provides numerous contexts for children to use their bodies to pretend when they practice the many poses that are named for animals and objects.

Emergent literacy

Emergent literacy refers to the reading and writing knowledge and skills that precede and lay the foundation for literacy. Yoga poses, breathing exercises, and meditations can easily be paired with the written word in order to increase phonological awareness, alphabet knowledge, and print awareness.

Appendix 2

Yoga Book Resources for Adults

Name	Author	Developmental domains
Yoga for Stuttering: Unifying the Voice, Breath, Mind & Body to Achieve Fluent Speech	Balakrishnan, J.M.	Breath support
YogaKids: Educating The Whole Child Through Yoga	Wenig, Marsha	Breath support, motor planning, vocabulary/concepts, symbolic play, emergent literacy
Yoga Therapy for Children with Autism and Special Needs	Goldberg, Louise	Communication, breath support, motor planning, vocabulary/concepts, symbolic play
Yoga for Children with Autism Spectrum Disorders: A Step-by-Step Guide for Parents and Caregivers	Betts, Dion E. and Betts, Stacey W.	Breath support, motor planning
Yoga for the Special Child: A Therapeutic Approach for Infants and Children with Down Syndrome, Cerebral Palsy, Autism Spectrum Disorders and Learning Disabilities	Sumar, Sonia	Breath support, motor planning
Yoga Therapy for Every Special Child: Meeting Needs in a Natural Setting	Williams, Nancy	Communication, breath support, motor planning, vocabulary/concepts, symbolic play

Learn with Yoga ABC Yoga Cards for Kids Instructor Guide	Ristuccia, Christine	Breath support, motor planning, vocabulary/concepts, symbolic play, emergent literacy
Storytime Yoga: Teaching Yoga to Children Through Story	Solis, Sydney	Breath support, emergent literacy
Yoga Games for Children: Fun and Fitness with Postures, Movements and Breath	Bersma, Danielle and Visscher, Marjoke	Communication, breath support, motor planning, vocabulary/concepts, symbolic play
Itsy Bitsy Yoga for Toddlers and Preschoolers: 8-Minute Routines to Help Your Child Grow Smarter, Be Happier, and Behave Better	Garabedian, Helen	Communication, breath support, motor planning, vocabulary/concepts, symbolic play, emergent literacy
Itsy Bitsy Yoga: Poses to Help Your Baby Sleep Longer, Digest Better, and Grow Stronger	Garabedian, Helen	Communication, breath support
Asanas for Autism and Special Needs: Yoga to Help Children with Their Emotions, Self-Regulation and Body Awareness	Hardy, Shawnee Thornton	Communication, breath support, motor planning, vocabulary/concepts
Create a Yoga Practice for Kids	Calhoun, Yael and Calhoun, Matthew R.	Communication, breath support, motor planning, vocabulary/concepts, symbolic play
Ready…Set… R.E.L.A.X.: A Research-Based Program of Relaxation, Learning, and Self-Esteem for Children	Allen, Jeffrey and Klein, Roger	Communication, breath support, motor planning, vocabulary/concepts symbolic play
Creative Yoga for Children: Inspiring the Whole Child Through Yoga, Songs, Literature, and Games	Rawlinson, Adrienne	Communication, breath support, motor planning, vocabulary/concepts, symbolic play, emergent literacy

cont.

Name	Author	Developmental domains
Yoga for Kids to Teens: Themes, Relaxation Techniques, Games, and an Introduction to SOLA Stikk Yoga	Calhoun, Matthew, Calhoun, Yael, and Hamory, Nicole	Communication, breath support, motor planning, vocabulary/concepts, symbolic play
Yoga for Children: 200+ Yoga Poses, Breathing Exercises, and Meditations for Healthier, Happier, More Resilient Children	Flynn, Lisa	Communication, breath support, motor planning, vocabulary/concepts, symbolic play, emergent literacy
The Yoga Zoo Adventure: Animal Poses and Games for Little Kids	Purperhart, Helen	Motor planning, vocabulary/concepts, symbolic play
Fly Like a Butterfly: Yoga for Children	Khalsa, Shakta Kaur	Breath support, vocabulary/concepts, symbolic play
Mindfulness and Yoga Skills for Children and Adolescents: 115 Activities for Trauma, Self-Regulation, Special Needs, and Anxiety	Neiman, Barbara	Breath support, motor planning, vocabulary/concepts, symbolic play
Little Flower Yoga for Kids	Harper, Jennifer Cohen	Breath support, motor planning, vocabulary/concepts, symbolic play
Yoga Calm for Children: Educating Heart, Mind, and Body	Gillen, Linea and Gillen, James	Communication, breath support
Baby Om: Yoga for Mothers and Babies	Staton, Laura and Perron, Sarah	Communication
Yoga Mama, Buddha Baby: The Workout for New Moms	Larson, Jyothi and Howard, Ken	Communication

Appendix 3

Yoga Book Resources for Children

Name	Author	Developmental domains
The ABCs of Yoga for Kids	Power, Teresa Anne	Vocabulary/concepts, symbolic play, emergent literacy
My Daddy Is a Pretzel: Yoga for Parents and Kids	Baptiste, Baron	Motor planning, vocabulary/concepts, symbolic play, emergent literacy
Learn with Yoga ABC Virtues	Ristuccia, Christine	Breath support, vocabulary/concepts, symbolic play, emergent literacy
Little Yoga: A Toddler's First Book of Yoga	Whitford, Rebecca	Vocabulary/concepts, symbolic play
Sleepy Little Yoga: A Toddler's Sleepy Book of Yoga	Whitford, Rebecca	Vocabulary/concepts, symbolic play
You Are a Lion! And Other Fun Yoga Poses	Yoo, Tae-Eun	Vocabulary/concepts, symbolic play, emergent literacy
Peaceful Piggy Meditation	MacLean, Kerry Lee	Vocabulary/concepts, emergent literacy
Peaceful Piggy Yoga	MacLean, Kerry Lee	Vocabulary/concepts, symbolic play, emergent literacy
Mindful Monkey, Happy Panda	Alderfer, Lauren and MacLean, Kerry Lee	Vocabulary/concepts, emergent literacy

cont.

Name	Author	Developmental domains
Babar's Yoga for Elephants	de Brunhoff, Laurent	Breath support, vocabulary/concepts, symbolic play, emergent literacy
Frog's Breathtaking Speech: How Children (and Frogs) Can Use Yoga Breathing to Deal with Anxiety, Anger and Tension	Chissick, Michael	Communication, breath support, motor planning, vocabulary/concepts, symbolic play, emergent literacy
Ladybird's Remarkable Relaxation: How Children (and Frogs, Dogs, Flamingos and Dragons) Can Use Yoga Relaxation to Help Deal with Stress, Grief, Bullying and Lack of Confidence	Chissick, Michael	Communication, breath support, vocabulary/concepts, emergent literacy
Seahorse's Magical Sun Sequences: How All Children (and Sea Creatures) Can Use Yoga to Feel Positive, Confident, and Completely Included	Chissick, Michael	Vocabulary/concepts, emergent literacy
Good Night, Animal World: A Kids Yoga Bedtime Story	Shardlow, Giselle	Vocabulary/concepts, symbolic play, emergent literacy
Hello, Bali: A Kids Yoga Island Adventure Book	Shardlow, Giselle	Vocabulary/concepts, symbolic play, emergent literacy
Rachel's Day in the Garden	Shardlow, Giselle	Vocabulary/concepts, symbolic play, emergent literacy

Sophia's Jungle Adventure	Shardlow, Giselle	Vocabulary/concepts, symbolic play, emergent literacy
I Love Yoga (Yoga for Kids)	Chryssicas, Mary Kaye	Communication, motor planning, vocabulary/concepts, symbolic play, literacy
Kids Yoga: Bedtime Rhymes	Maier, Jeff	Vocabulary/concepts, symbolic play, emergent literacy
The Kids' Yoga Book of Feelings	Humphrey, Mary	Communication, vocabulary/concepts, symbolic play, literacy
I Can't Believe It's Yoga for Kids!	Trivell, Lisa	Vocabulary/concepts, symbolic play, literacy
Yoga for Kids: Ashok Wahi's the Missing Peace	Wahi, Ashok, Monroe, Miriam, and Pappas, Stefani	Vocabulary/concepts, symbolic play, literacy
Breathe, Chill: A Handy Book of Games and Techniques Introducing Breathing, Meditation and Relaxation to Kids and Teens	Roberts, Lisa	Breath support, vocabulary/concepts, literacy
Dogi the Yogi	Scrivan, Maria Notarlie	Vocabulary/concepts, symbolic play, emergent literacy
Bal Yoga for Kids	Kacev, Glenda and Roth, Sylvia	Vocabulary/concepts, symbolic play, emergent literacy
Good Morning Yoga	Gates, Mariam	Breath support, vocabulary/concepts
Good Night Yoga	Gates, Mariam	Breath support, vocabulary/concepts
I Am Yoga	Verde, Susan	Vocabulary/concepts, symbolic play
Adam's Yoga Journey	Preiss, Anat	Communication, breath support, vocabulary/concepts, symbolic play
Yoga for Busy Little Hands	Danzig, Marsha Therese	Communication, motor planning, vocabulary/concepts, symbolic play, emergent literacy
Breathe	Magoon, Scott	Breath support, vocabulary/concepts

Appendix 4

Yoga Card Deck Resources

Name	Author/ publisher/ company	Developmental domains
The Kids' Yoga Deck: 50 Poses and Games	Buckley, Annie	Communication, breath support, vocabulary/ concepts, symbolic play, emergent literacy
Yoga Pretzels	Guber, Tara and Kalish, Leah	Communication, breath support, vocabulary/ concepts, symbolic play, emergent literacy
Yoga Planet	Guber, Tara and Kalish, Leah	Communication, breath support, vocabulary/ concepts, symbolic play, emergent literacy
Body Poetry: Yoga Cards	Roylco	Vocabulary/concepts, symbolic play
Learn with Yoga: ABC Yoga Cards for Kids	Ristuccia, Christine	Breath support, motor planning, vocabulary/ concepts, symbolic play, emergent literacy
Little Lotus Kid's Yoga Cards	Johnson, Tracy	Communication, breath support, motor planning, vocabulary/concepts, symbolic play, emergent literacy
Wai Lana's Little Yogis: Game Cards	Lana, Wai	Communication, breath support, vocabulary/ concepts, symbolic play, emergent literacy

Wai Lana's Little Yogis: Daydream Game Cards	Lana, Wai	Communication, breath support, vocabulary/ concepts, symbolic play, emergent literacy
Wai Lana's Little Yogis: Fun Songs Game Cards	Lana, Wai	Communication, breath support, motor planning, vocabulary/concepts, symbolic play, emergent literacy
Yogarilla: Exercises and Activities	Super Duper Publications	Communication, breath support, vocabulary/ concepts, symbolic play, emergent literacy
ABCs for Little Yogis: Bhakti Yoga Flash Cards	Nonino, Lauren	Vocabulary/concepts, emergent literacy
The ABCs of Yoga for Kids: 56 Learning Cards	Power, Teresa Anne	Vocabulary/concepts, symbolic play, emergent literacy
Yoga 4 Classrooms	Flynn, Lisa	Breath support, vocabulary/ concepts, symbolic play, emergent literacy
Self-Regulation Flash Cards	Move with Me: Yoga Adventures	Breath support, motor planning, vocabulary/ concepts, symbolic play, emergent literacy
The YogaKids Tool Box	YogaKids	Communication, breath support, motor planning, vocabulary/concepts, symbolic play, emergent literacy
Good Night, Animal World Yoga Cards	Kids Yoga Stories	Vocabulary/concepts, symbolic play, emergent literacy
Yoga Poses for Kids Cards	Kids Yoga Stories	Vocabulary/concepts, symbolic play, emergent literacy
Magical Moves	Aldersey-Williams, Justine	Vocabulary/concepts, symbolic play, emergent literacy

cont.

Name	Author/ publisher/ company	Developmental domains
Angel Bear Yoga: A Pose a Day Play Deck	Eley, Christi	Communication, breath support, motor planning, vocabulary/concepts, symbolic play, emergent literacy
Creative Yoga Games for Kids	Reinhardt, Edna	Communication, vocabulary/ concepts, symbolic play, emergent literacy
I Am Yogi Twist Flash Cards	Aziam Books	Communication, vocabulary/ concepts, symbolic play, emergent literacy

Appendix 5

Yoga Game Resources

Name	Creator/company	Developmental domains
Yoga Spinner Game	Thinkfun	Communication, vocabulary/concepts, symbolic play, emergent literacy
Memory Yoga	Thinkfun	Communication, vocabulary/concepts
Yoga Cards the Game	Thinkfun	Communication, vocabulary/concepts, symbolic play, emergent literacy
Stress Quest	Dubow, Jennifer	Communication, vocabulary/concepts, emergent literacy
The Magic Path of Yoga	Upside Down Games	Communication, vocabulary/concepts, symbolic play, emergent literacy
The Yoga Garden Game	YogaKids	Communication, vocabulary/concepts, symbolic play, emergent literacy
Yoga-Yingo Classic Set	Yoga-Yingo	Communication, vocabulary/concepts, symbolic play
Memo Yoga	Upside Down Games	Communication, vocabulary/concepts
Yogi Finders	Upside Down Games	Communication, vocabulary/concepts
Yogi Cards	Upside Down Games	Communication, vocabulary/concepts, symbolic play, emergent literacy

cont.

Name	Creator/company	Developmental domains
Yoga Match: A Memory and Movement Card Game	Light Connections Press	Communication, vocabulary/concepts, symbolic play, emergent literacy
MagneTalk Yogarilla: Exercises & Activities Magnetic Board Game	Super Duper Publications	Communication, vocabulary/concepts, symbolic play, emergent literacy
YogaMe ABC	Janod	Communication, vocabulary/concepts, emergent literacy
YogaMe Zoo	Janod	Communication, vocabulary/concepts, symbolic play
Turasa: A Yoga Adventure	Turasa Yoga	Communication, vocabulary/concepts, symbolic play, emergent literacy

Appendix 6

Yoga CD Resources

Name	Artist/label	Developmental domains
Wai Lana's Little Yogis: Daydream	Lana, Wai	Vocabulary/concepts
Angel Bear Yoga: Adventure Stories—Creative Visualizations for Relaxation, Reflection and Quiet Time	Eley, Christi	Vocabulary/concepts
Yoga for Kids	Great Lake Sports	Breath support, vocabulary/concepts, symbolic play
Come Play Yoga!	Karma Kids Yoga	Motor planning, vocabulary/concepts, symbolic play
Dance for the Sun: Yoga Songs for Kids	Willey, Kira	Breath support, motor planning, vocabulary/concepts, symbolic play
Kings & Queens of the Forest: Yoga Songs for Kids Vol. 2	Willey, Kira	Breath support, vocabulary/concepts, symbolic play
How to Be a Cloud: Yoga Songs for Kids Vol. 3	Willey, Kira	Breath support, vocabulary/concepts, symbolic play
Yoga Child: A Peaceful Place Inside	The Bingo Kids	Breath support, motor planning, vocabulary/concepts, symbolic play, emergent literacy
Musical Yoga Adventures	Lara, Linda	Vocabulary/concepts, symbolic play

cont.

Name	Artist/label	Developmental domains
Musical Yoga Adventures: World Journey	Lara, Linda	Communication, motor planning, vocabulary/concepts, symbolic play
Namaste! Songs, Yoga & Meditations for Young Yogis!	Carbone, Christopher	Breath support, motor planning, vocabulary/concepts, symbolic play
Still Quiet Place: Mindfulness for Young Children	Saltzman, Amy	Breath support, vocabulary/concepts, symbolic play
I Grow with Yoga: Yoga Songs for Children	Haynes, Sammie and Flynn, Lisa	Breath support, vocabulary/concepts, symbolic play
Happy Little Hearts: Health & Healing Meditations for Children	Cavanough, Katrina	Breath support, vocabulary/concepts
Radiant Child Music: Happy	Khalsa, Shakta Kaur with Clarke, Alima Dyal	Vocabulary/concepts, symbolic play
Radiant Child Music: Cozy	Khalsa, Shakta Kaur with Clarke, Alima Dyal	Vocabulary/concepts, symbolic play
Children's Yoga Songs for the Classroom	Kelbach, Darlene and Popielski, Matthew	Breath support, vocabulary/concepts, symbolic play, emergent literacy
Yoga Lounge	Putumayo World Music	Motor planning
Yoga Nidra for Kids of All Ages	Gretz, Emily with Wolf, Steve	Breath support, vocabulary/concepts
The Children's School of Yoga: Hello and Goodbye Chants for Children Under Age 5	The Children's School of Yoga	Communication, breath support, vocabulary/concepts
Tommy & Tina's Yoga Fun: Sing Along Yoga Rhymes	Sutton, Lindsey and Cordes, Rebecca	Breath support, motor planning, vocabulary/concepts, symbolic play, emergent literacy
StoryBook Yoga	Lederer, Susan Hendler	Vocabulary/concepts, symbolic play, emergent literacy
Kidding Around Yoga: Music for Little Yogis	Kidding Around Yoga	Motor planning, vocabulary/concepts, symbolic play

Appendix 7

Yoga DVD Resources

Name	Creator/ company	Developmental domains
Kids World Yoga	Van Block, Bridget	Communication, breath support, vocabulary/concepts
Yoga for Children with Special Needs	Baskauskas, Aras and Collins, Britt	Breath support, vocabulary/concepts
YogaKids: For Ages 3–6	Gaiam	Breath support, vocabulary/concepts
YogaKids 2: ABCs for Ages 3–6	Gaiam	Vocabulary/concepts, symbolic play, emergent literacy
YogaKids 3: Silly to Calm for Ages 3–6	Gaiam	Breath support, vocabulary/concepts
Kidding Around Yoga: Learn & Practice Yoga	Kidding Around Yoga	Breath support, vocabulary/ concepts, symbolic play
Scooter & Me: The Magic Scooter	Move with Me: Yoga Adventures	Vocabulary/concepts, symbolic play, emergent literacy
Scooter & Me: Monkeying Around at the Zoo	Move with Me: Yoga Adventures	Vocabulary/concepts, symbolic play
Scooter & Me: Possum's Tail	Move with Me: Yoga Adventures	Vocabulary/concepts, symbolic play
Scooter & Me: Active Play and Social Skills Program	Move with Me: Yoga Adventures	Communication, vocabulary/ concepts, symbolic play, emergent literacy
Yoga Motion	Namaste Kid	Breath support, vocabulary/ concepts, symbolic play
Once Upon a Mat	Namaste Kid	Breath support, vocabulary/ concepts, symbolic play

cont.

Name	Creator/ company	Developmental domains
Sport Yoga	Namaste Kid	Breath support, vocabulary/ concepts, symbolic play
Storyland Yoga	Playful Planet	Communication, vocabulary/ concepts, symbolic play
Yoga Journal's Family Yoga with Rodney Yee, Donna Fone, & Kids	Gaiam	Communication, breath support, vocabulary/concepts
Wai Lana's Little Yogis: Volumes 1 & 2	Lana, Wai	Breath support, vocabulary/ concepts, symbolic play
Wai Lana's Little Yogis: Fun Songs Cartoon	Lana, Wai	Vocabulary/concepts, symbolic play
Wai Lana's Little Yogis: Daydream	Lana, Wai	Vocabulary/concepts
Yoga for Families	Bayview Entertainment/ Widowmaker	Communication, breath support, vocabulary/concepts
Yoga Skills for Youth Peacemakers	Shanti Generation, LLC	Breath support, vocabulary/concepts
Yoga	BeeTwixt	Vocabulary/concepts
Sing Song Yoga	Sing Song Yoga	Vocabulary/concepts, symbolic play
Happy Yoga with Sarah Starr: Children's Yoga and Zoo Animals	Sarah Starr	Breath support, vocabulary/ concepts, symbolic play
A Child's Way to Yoga: Introducing Children to Yoga Through Movement and Music	Hal's Digital Mojo, Inc.	Vocabulary/concepts, symbolic play
Cosmic Kids! Yoga	Cosmic Kids Yoga	Vocabulary/concepts, symbolic play
Yoga to Go for Kids!	Face Productions	Breath support, vocabulary/ concepts, symbolic play

Kids Yoga with Phonics	Little Sensei	Vocabulary/concepts, symbolic play, emergent literacy
Yoga for the Kid in All of Us	Yogamazing	Vocabulary/concepts, symbolic play
Yoga for Children with Vasanthi Bhat and Students	Vasantha Yoga	Vocabulary/concepts, symbolic play
Lazy Lizards Yoga for Kids!	Lazy Lizards Yoga	Vocabulary/concepts, symbolic play
Family Acro Yoga	Van Block, Bridget	Communication, vocabulary/concepts
Yoga with Danielle Rae on the Farm	Rae, Danielle	Breath support, vocabulary/concepts, symbolic play
Yoga Adventures with Down Dog: A Yoga Alphabet Play Date	Power, Teresa Anne	Vocabulary/concepts, symbolic play, emergent literacy
Yoga for Children with Developmental Challenges	Flynn, Mary	Breath support, vocabulary/concepts
Itsy Bitsy Yoga: Play n' Flourish	Itsy Bitsy Yoga International	Communication, vocabulary/concepts
Manga Yoga Cherry Blossom	Lichtung Media Ltd.	Breath support, vocabulary/concepts, symbolic play

Appendix 8

Yoga Web-Based Resources

Website	Author	Link and developmental domains
OMazing Kids	Moorad, Angela	http://omazingkidsllc.com/about Communication, breath support, motor planning, vocabulary/concepts, symbolic play, emergent literacy
Cosmic Kids	Amor, Jaime	www.cosmickids.com/about Communication, breath support, motor planning, vocabulary/concepts, symbolic play, emergent literacy
The Kids Yoga Resource	Flynn, Lisa	www.thekidsyogaresource.com Communication, breath support, motor planning, vocabulary/concepts, symbolic play, emergent literacy
Yoga Kids	Wenig, Marsha	http://yogakids.com Communication, breath support, motor planning, vocabulary/concepts, symbolic play, emergent literacy
Karma Kids Yoga	Vilchez-Blatt, Shari	www.karmakidsyoga.com Communication, breath support, motor planning, vocabulary/concepts, symbolic play, emergent literacy
Little Flower Yoga	Harper, Jennifer Cohen	http://littlefloweryoga.com Communication, breath support, motor planning, vocabulary/concepts, symbolic play, emergent literacy
Kids Yoga Stories	Shardlow, Giselle	www.kidsyogastories.com Vocabulary/concepts, symbolic play, emergent literacy

Yoga for the Special Child	Sumar, Sonia	www.specialyoga.com
		Breath support
GoGo Babies	Skove, Ellyne	www.gogobabies.net
		Communication
Lil Omm Yoga	Siliki, Pleasance	http://lilomm.com/book
		Communication, vocabulary/concepts

References

Adams, M.J. (1990) *Beginning to Read: Thinking and Learning about Print.* Cambridge, MA: MIT Press.

Alkalay, D. (2001) *Meditation: A Practitioner's Handbook.* Rego Park, NY: The Genesis Society, Inc.

American Psychiatric Association (2013) *Diagnostic and Statistical Manual of Mental Disorders, 5th edition (DSM-5).* Washington, DC: Author.

American Speech-Language-Hearing Association (ASHA) (2007) *Childhood Apraxia of Speech.* Rockville, MD: American Speech-Language-Hearing Association. Available at www.asha.org/policy/TR2007-00278/, accessed on 21 November 2016.

Ayres, A.J. (1995) *Sensory Integration and the Child.* Los Angeles, CA: Western Psychological Services.

Bagui, S. (1998) "Reasons for increased learning using multimedia." *Journal of Educational Multimedia and Hypermedia 7*, 1, 3–18.

Balakrishnan, J.M. (2009) *Yoga for Stuttering: Unifying the Voice, Breath, Mind and Body to Achieve Fluent Speech.* Berkeley, CA: North Atlantic Books.

Baron-Cohen, S., Wheelwright, S., Lawson, J., Griffin, R. *et al.* (2005) "Empathizing and Systematizing in Autism Spectrum Conditions." In F.R. Volkmar, R. Paul, A. Klin, and D. Cohen (eds) *Handbook on Autism and Pervasive Developmental Disorders: Diagnosis, Development, Neurobiology, and Behavior Volume I, 3rd Edition.* Hoboken, NJ: John Wiley & Sons, Inc.

Bates, E., Marchman, V., Thal, D., Fenson, L. *et al.* (1994) "Developmental and stylistic variation in the composition of early vocabulary." *Journal of Child Language 21*, 1, 85–123.

Bauman-Waengler, J. (2012) *Articulatory and Phonological Impairments: A Clinical Focus, 4th Edition.* Boston, MA: Pearson Education, Inc.

Bauminger-Zviely, N. (2014) "School-age Children with ASD." In F.R. Volkmar, S.J. Rogers, R. Paul, and K.A. Pelfrey (eds) *Handbook on Autism and Pervasive Developmental Disorders: Diagnosis, Development, and Brain Mechanisms Volume I, 4th Edition.* Hoboken, NJ: John Wiley & Sons, Inc.

Bell, N. (1991) "Gestalt imagery: a critical factor in language comprehension." *Annals of Dyslexia 41*, 1, 246–260.

Bell, N. (2007) *Visualizing and Verbalizing for Language Comprehension and Thinking, 2nd Edition*. San Luis Obispo, CA: Gander Publishing.

Bersma, D. and Visscher, M. (2003) *Yoga Games for Children: Fun and Fitness with Postures, Movements and Breath*. Alameda, CA: Hunter House Inc.

Betts, D. and Betts, S.W. (2006) *Yoga for Children with Autism Spectrum Disorders: A Step-by-Step Guide for Parents and Caregivers*. London: Jessica Kingsley Publishers.

Biemiller, A. (2005) "Size and Sequence in Vocabulary Development: Implications for Choosing Words for Primary Grade Vocabulary Instruction." In E.H. Hiebert and M. Kamil (eds) *Teaching and Learning Vocabulary: Bringing Research to Practice*. Mahwah, NY: Erlbaum.

Birdee, G.S., Yeh, G., Wayne, P.M., Phillips, R.S., Davis, R.B., and Gardiner, P. (2009) "Clinical applications to yoga for the pediatric population: A systematic review." *Academic Pediatrics 9*, 4, 212–220.

Black, L.I., Clarke, T.C., Barnes, P.M., Stussman, B.J., and Nahin, R.L. (2015) "Use of complementary health approaches among children aged 4–17 years in the United States: National health interview survey, 2007–2012." *National Health Statistics Reports 78*, 1–18.

Bleile, K.M. (2004) *Manual of Articulation and Phonological Disorders: Infancy Through Adulthood, 2nd Edition*. Clifton Park, NY: Delmar Cengage Learning.

Bloom, L. and Lahey, M. (1978) *Language Development and Language Disorders*. New York, NY: Macmillan.

Bloom, L. and Tinker, E. (2001) "The intentionality model and language acquisition." *Monographs of the Society for Research in Child Development 66*, 4, Serial No. 267.

Boliek, C.A., Hixon, T.J., Watson, P.J., and Jones, P.B. (2009) "Refinement of speech breathing in healthy 4- to 6-year-old children." *Journal of Speech, Language, and Hearing Research 52*, 4, 990–1007.

Boyle, C.A., Boulet, S., Schieve, L., Cohen, R.A. *et al.* (2011) "Trends in the prevalence of developmental disabilities in U.S. children, 1997–2008." *Pediatrics 127*, 6, 1034–1042.

Boyle, M.P. (2011) "Mindfulness training in stuttering therapy: A tutorial for speech-language pathologists." *Journal of Fluency Disorders 36*, 2, 122–129.

Broad, W.J. (2012) *The Science of Yoga: The Risks and the Rewards*. New York, NY: Simon & Schuster Paperbacks.

Brulé, D. (2017) *Just Breathe: Mastering Breathwork for Success in Life, Love, Business, and Beyond*. New York: Atria/Enliven Books. Website: www.breathmastery. com.

Bruner, J. (1983) *Child Talk*. New York: W.W. Norton and Company.

Butzer, B., Day, D., Potts, A., Ryan C. *et al.* (2015) "Effects of a classroom-based yoga intervention on cortisol and behavior in second- and third-grade students: A pilot study." *Journal of Evidenced-Based Complementary Alternative Medicine 20*, 1, 41–49.

Centers for Disease Control and Prevention, Division of Birth Defects, National Center on Birth Defects and Developmental Disabilities (2016) *Autism Spectrum Disorder: Data and Statistics.* Atlanta, GA: Centers for Disease Control and Prevention. Available at www.cdc.gov/ncbddd/autism/data.html, accessed on 11 July 2016.

Clark, J.M. and Paivio, A. (1991) "Dual coding theory and education." *Educational Psychology Review 3,* 3, 149–210.

Coplan, J. and Gleason, J.R. (1988) "Unclear speech: Recognition and significance of unintelligible speech in preschool children." *Pediatrics 82,* 3, 447–452.

Crais, E., Douglas, D., and Campbell, C. (2004) "The intersection of the development of gestures and intentionality." *Journal of Speech, Language, and Hearing Research 47,* 3, 678–694.

Cuomo, N. (2007) *Integrated Yoga: Yoga with a Sensory Integrative Approach.* London: Jessica Kingsley Publishers.

Dore, J. (1975) "Holophrases, speech acts, and language universals." *Journal of Child Language 2,* 20–40.

Duffy, J.R. (2012) *Motor Speech Disorders: Substrates, Differential Diagnosis, and Management, 3rd Edition.* St. Louis, MO: Elsevier Mosby.

Eggleston, B. (2015) "The benefits of yoga for children in schools." *The International Journal of Health, Wellness, and Society 5,* 3, 1–7.

Ehleringer, J. (2010) "Yoga for children on the autism spectrum." *International Journal of Yoga Therapy 20,* 1, 131–139.

Ellis, M.J. (1973) *Why People Play.* Englewood Cliffs, NJ: Prentice Hall.

Flipsen Jr., P. (2006) "Measuring the intelligibility of conversational speech in children." *Clinical Linguistics and Phonetics 20,* 4, 303–312.

Flook, L., Smalley, S.L., Kitil, M.J., Galla, B.M. *et al.* (2010) "Effects of mindful awareness practices on executive functions in elementary school children." *Journal of Applied School Psychology 26,* 1, 70–95.

Flynn, L. (2013) *Yoga for Children.* Avon, MA: Adams Media.

Flynn, L. and Ebert, M. (2013) "Bringing yoga to the classroom: Tools for learning, skills for life." *Yoga Therapy Today, Summer,* 24–27.

Galantino, M.L., Galbavy, R., and Quinn, L. (2008) "Therapeutic effects of yoga for children: A systematic review of the literature." *Pediatric Physical Therapy 20,* 1, 66–80.

Garabedian, H. (2004) *Itsy Bitsy Yoga: Poses to Help Your Baby Sleep Longer, Digest Better, and Grow Stronger.* New York, NY: Simon and Schuster.

Garabedian, H. (2008) *Itsy Bitsy Yoga for Toddlers and Preschoolers: 8-Minute Routines to Help Your Child Grow Smarter, Be Happier, and Behave Better.* Cambridge, MA: Da Capo Press.

Gates, B. (2010) "Keynote address to the Creating Digital Dividends Conference." Available at voicesofdemocracy.umd.edu/gates-keynote-address-speech-text, accessed on 09 February 2017.

Gerber, S. and Prizant, B.M. (2000) "Speech, Language, and Intervention Assessment and Intervention for Children." In *Clinical Practice Guidelines: Interdisciplinary Council on Development and Learning Disorders*. Bethesda, MD: The Interdisciplinary Council on Development and Learning, Inc.

Gerber, S. and Wankoff, L. (2014) "Historical and Contemporary Views of the Nature-Nurture Debate: A Continuum of Perspectives for the Speech-Language Pathologist." In N. Capone Singleton and B.B. Shulman (eds) *Language Development: Foundations, Processes, and Clinical Applications, 2nd Edition*. Burlington, MA: Jones and Bartlett Learning.

Giess, S. (2014) "Early Transitions: Literacy Development in the Emergent Literacy and Early Literacy Stages." In N. Capone Singleton and B.B. Shulman (eds) *Language Development: Foundations, Processes, and Clinical Applications, 2nd Edition*. Burlington, MA: Jones and Bartlett Learning.

Gilman, M. (2014) *Body and Voice: Somatic Re-education*. San Diego, CA: Plural Publishing.

Goldberg, L. (2013) *Yoga Therapy for Children with Autism and Special Needs*. New York, NY: W.W. Norton and Co.

Goldfield, B.A., Snow, C.E., and Willenberg, I.A. (2017) "Variation in Language Development: Implications for Theory and Research." In J. Berko Gleason and N. Bernstein Ratner (eds) *The Development of Language, 9th Edition*. Boston, MA: Pearson.

Greater Good Science Center, University of California, Berkeley (n.d.) *What Is Mindfulness?* Berkeley, CA: Greater Good Science Center, University of California, Berkeley. Available at http://greatergood.berkeley.edu/topic/mindfulness/definition, accessed on 21 November 2016.

Greenspan, S.I. (1985) *First Feelings*. New York, NY: Viking Press.

Halliday, M.A.K. (1975) *Learning How to Mean: Explorations in the Development of Language*. London, UK: Edward Arnold Publishers Ltd.

Hamaguchi, P. (2010) *Childhood Speech, Language and Listening Problems, 3rd Edition*. Hoboken, NJ: John Wiley & Sons, Inc.

Hardy, S.T. (2015) *Asanas for Autism and Special Needs: Yoga to Help Children with Their Emotions, Self-Regulation and Body Awareness*. London, UK: Jessica Kingsley Publishers.

Harper, J.C. (2010) "Teaching yoga in urban elementary schools." *International Journal of Yoga Therapy 20*, 99–109.

Heath, S.B. and Street, B.V. (2008) *On Ethnography: Approaches to Language and Literacy Research*. New York, NY: Teachers College Press.

Hixon, T.J. and Hoit, J.D. (2005) *Evaluation and Management of Speech Breathing Disorders: Principles and Methods*. Tucson, AZ: Redington Brown LLC.

Hupbach, A., Gomez, R.L., Bootzin, R.R., and Nadel, L. (2009) "Nap-dependent learning in infants." *Developmental Science 12*, 6, 1007–1012.

Hyde, A.M. (2012) "The Yoga in Schools Movement: Using Standards for Educating the Whole Child and Making Space for Teacher Self-Care." In J.A. Gorlewski, B. Porfilio, and D.A. Gorlewski (eds) *Using Standards and High Stakes Testing for Students: Exploiting Power with Critical Pedagogy.* New York, NY: Peter Lang Publishing, Inc.

Jensen, P.S. and Kenny, D.T. (2004) "The effects of yoga on the attention and behavior of boys with Attention-Deficit/Hyperactivity Disorder (ADHD)." *Journal of Attention Disorders 7*, 4, 205–216.

Johnston, J. and Wong, M.Y. (2002) "Cultural differences in beliefs and practices concerning talk to children." *Journal of Speech, Language, and Hearing Research 45*, 5, 916–926.

Justice, L.M. and Pence, K.L. (2005) *Scaffolding with Storybooks: A Guide for Enhancing Young Children's Language and Literacy Achievement.* Newark, DE: International Reading Association.

Kaley-Isley, L.C., Peterson, J., Fischer, C., and Peterson, E. (2010) "Yoga as a complementary therapy for children and adolescents: A guide for clinicians." *Psychiatry 7*, 8, 20–32.

Kasari, C. and Chang, Y. (2014) "Play Development in Children with Autism Spectrum Disorders: Skills, Object Play, and Interventions." In F.R. Volkmar, S.J. Rogers, R. Paul, and K.A. Pelfrey (eds) *Handbook on Autism and Pervasive Developmental Disorders: Diagnosis, Development, and Brain Mechanisms Volume I, 4th Edition.* Hoboken, NJ: John Wiley & Sons, Inc.

Kauffman, H., Hallperin, W., Molden, B., and Klein, E. (2010) *Yoga: An Alternative Method in Stuttering Treatment.* Poster presented at the Annual Convention of the American Speech-Language-Hearing Association, Philadelphia, PA.

Kenny, M. (2002) "Integrative movement therapy™: Yoga-based therapy as a viable and effective intervention for autism and related disorders." *International Journal of Yoga Therapy 12*, 71–79.

Kim, S.H., Paul, R., Tager-Flusberg, H., and Lord, C. (2014) "Language and Communication in Autism." In F.R. Volkmar, S.J. Rogers, R. Paul, and K.A. Pelfrey (eds) *Handbook on Autism and Pervasive Developmental Disorders: Diagnosis, Development, and Brain Mechanisms Volume I, 4th Edition.* Hoboken, NJ: John Wiley & Sons, Inc.

Koenig, K.P., Buckley-Reen, A., and Garg, S. (2012) "Efficacy of the Get Ready to Learn yoga program among children with autism spectrum disorders: A pretest-posttest control group design." *American Journal of Occupational Therapy 66*, 5, 538–546.

Lahey, M. (1988) *Language Disorders and Language Development.* New York, NY: Macmillan Publishing Company.

Larson, J. and Howard, K. (2002) *Yoga Mom, Buddha Baby: The Yoga Workout for New Moms.* New York, NY: Bantam Books.

Law, J., Boyle, J., Harris, F., Harkness, A., and Nye, C. (2000) "Prevalence and natural history of primary speech and language delay: Findings from a systematic review of the literature." *International Journal of Language and Communication Disorders 35*, 2, 165–188.

Lederer, S. (2012) "Storybook Yoga: Integrating Shared Book Reading and Yoga to Nurture the Whole Child." In R. Goldfarb (ed.) *Translational Speech-Language Pathology and Audiology.* San Diego, CA: Plural Publishing.

Lee, L. (2006) "Enhancing balance, lower extremity function, and gait in people with Parkinson's disease through yoga exercise." *American Journal of Physical Medicine and Rehabilitation 85*, 3, 284.

Leonard, L.B. (2014) *Children with Specific Language Impairment.* Cambridge, MA: MIT Press.

Love, R.J. (2000) *Childhood Motor Speech Disability, 2nd Edition.* Needham Heights, MA: Allyn and Bacon.

McCall, T. (2007) *Yoga as Medicine: The Yogic Prescription for Health and Healing.* New York, NY: Bantam Dell.

Melzi, G. and Schick, A.R. (2017) "Language and Literacy in the School Years." In J. Berko Gleason and N. Bernstein Ratner (eds) *The Development of Language, 9th Edition.* Boston, MA: Pearson.

Miller, J. and Paul, R. (1995) *The Clinical Assessment of Language Comprehension.* Baltimore, MD: Brookes Publishing Co.

Milosky, L.M. (1994) "Nonliteral Language Abilities: Seeing the Forest for the Trees." In G.P. Wallach and K.G. Butler (eds) *Language Learning Disabilities in School-Age Children and Adolescents.* Needham Heights, MA: Allyn and Bacon.

Nagy, W.E. and Scott, J.A. (2000) "Vocabulary processes." In M.L. Kamil, P.B. Mosenthal, P.D. Pearson, and R. Barr (eds) *Handbook of Reading Research, Volume 3.* Mahwah, NJ: Erlbaum.

National Institute on Deafness and Other Communication Disorders (2010) *Statistics on Voice, Speech, and Language.* Bethesda, MD: National Institute on Deafness and Other Communication Disorders. Available at www.nidcd.nih.gov/health/statistics/pages/vsl.aspx, accessed on 21 November 2016.

Nelson, K. (1973) "Structure and strategy in learning to talk." *Monographs of the Society for Research in Child Development 38*, Serial No. 149.

Newman, R. and Sachs, J. (2017) "Communication Development in Infancy." In J. Berko Gleason and N. Bernstein Ratner (eds) *The Development of Language, 9th Edition.* Boston, MA: Pearson.

Nippold, M.A. (2007) *Later Language Development: School-Age Children, Adolescents, and Young Adults, 3rd Edition.* Austin, TX: ProEd.

O'Sullivan, S.B. and Schmitz, T.J. (2001) *Physical Rehabilitation: Assessment and Treatment.* Philadelphia, PA: F.A. Davis Company.

Parten, M.B. (1932) "Social participation among preschool children." *Journal of Abnormal and Social Psychology 27*, 3, 243–269.

Paul, R. and Norbury, C.F. (2012) *Language Disorders from Infancy Through Adolescence.* St. Louis, MO: Elsevier Mosby.

Pence Turnbull, K.L. and Justice, L.M. (2017) *Language Development: From Theory to Practice, 3rd Edition.* Upper Saddle River, NJ: Pearson.

Pepper, J. and Weitzman, E. (2004) *It Takes Two to Talk.* Toronto, CA: The Hanen Centre.

Piaget, J. (1962) *Play, Dreams, and Imitation in Childhood.* New York, NY: W.W. Norton and Company.

Premack, D. and Woodruff, G. (1978) "Does the chimpanzee have a theory of mind?" *Behavioral and Brain Sciences 1,* 4, 515–526.

Pullen, P.C. and Justice, L.M. (2003) "Enhancing phonological awareness, print awareness, and oral language skills in preschool children." *Intervention in School and Clinic 39,* 2, 87–98.

Rawlinson, A. (2013) *Creative Yoga for Children: Inspiring the Whole Child Through Yoga, Songs, Literature, and Games.* Berkeley, CA: North Atlantic Books.

Restak, R.M. and Grubin, D. (2001) *The Secret Life of the Brain.* Washington, DC: National Academies Press.

Rich, N.C. (2005) "Levels of evidence." *Journal of Women's Health Physical Therapy 29,* 2, 19–20.

Ristuccia, C. (2010) *Learn with Yoga: ABC Yoga Cards for Kids Instructor's Guide.* Tybee Island, GA: Addriya Yoga, LLC.

Satchidananda, S. (2011) *The Yoga Sutras of Patanjali.* Buckingham, VA: Integral Yoga Publications.

Saville-Troike, M. (2003) *The Ethnography of Communication: An Introduction, 3rd Edition.* Oxford, UK: Blackwell Publishing Ltd.

Schickendanz, J.A. and Collins, M.F. (2013) *So Much More than the ABCs: The Early Phases of Reading and Writing.* Washington, DC: National Association for the Education of Young Children.

Seikel, J.A., King, D.W., and Drumright, D.G. (2000) *Anatomy and Physiology for Speech, Language, and Hearing.* San Diego, CA: Singular Publishing Group.

Serwacki, M.L. and Cook-Cottone, C. (2012) "Yoga in the schools: A systematic review of the literature." *International Journal of Yoga Therapy 22,* 1, 101–110.

Shipley, K.G. and McAfee, J.G. (2009) *Assessment in Speech-Language Pathology: A Resource Manual, 4th Edition.* New York, NY: Delmar Cengage Learning.

Shonkoff, J. and Phillips, D. (eds) (2000) *From Neurons to Neighborhoods: The Science of Early Childhood Development.* Washington, DC: National Academy Press.

Simpkins, A.M. and Simpkins, C.A. (2011) *Meditation and Yoga in Psychotherapy.* Hoboken, NJ: John Wiley & Sons, Inc.

Solis, S. (2006) *Storytime Yoga™: Teaching Yoga to Children Through Story.* Boulder, CO: The Mythic Yoga Studio, LLC.

Stein, N. and Glenn, C. (1979) "An Analysis of Story Comprehension in Elementary School Children." In R. Freedle (ed.) *New Directions in Discourse Processing, Volume II.* Norwood, NJ: Ablex.

Stern, D. (1985) *The Interpersonal World of the Infant.* New York, NY: Basic Books.

Sumar, S. (1998) *Yoga for the Special Child.* Sarasota, FL: Special Yoga Publications.

Tarullo, A.R., Balsam, P.D., and Fifer, W.P. (2011) "Sleep and infant learning." *Infant and Child Development 20,* 1, 35–46.

Taylor, O. (1999) "Cultural Issues and Language Acquisition." In O. Taylor and L. Leonard (eds) *Language Acquisition Across North America*. San Diego, CA: Singular.

Teale, W.H. and Sulzby, E. (1986) "Emergent Literacy as a Perspective for Examining How Children Become Writers and Readers." In W.H. Teale and E. Sulzby (eds) *Emergent Literacy: Writing and Reading*. Norwood, NJ: Ablex.

Thygeson, M.V., Hooke, M.C., Clapsaddle, J., Robbins, A., and Moquist, K. (2010) "Peaceful play yoga: Serenity and balance for children with cancer and their parents." *Journal of Pediatric Oncology Nursing 27*, 5, 276–284.

Tobey, E.A. and Rampp, D.L. (1987) "Neurological correlates of speech." In M.I. Gottlieb and J.E. Williams (eds) *Textbook of Developmental Pediatrics*. New York, NY: Plenum Publishing Corporation.

Tomblin, J.B., Records, N.L., Buckwalter, P., Zhang, X., Smith, E., and O'Brien, M. (1997) "Prevalence of specific language impairment in kindergarten children." *Journal of Speech, Language, and Hearing Research 40*, 6, 1245–1260.

Uccelli, P., Rowe, M.L., and Pan, B.A. (2017) "Semantic Development: Learning the Meanings of Words." In J. Berko Gleason and N. Bernstein Ratner (eds) *The Development of Language, 9th Edition*. Boston, MA: Pearson.

United Nations Educational, Scientific and Cultural Organization (2004) *The Plurality of Literacy and Its Implications for Policies and Programmes: Position Paper*. France: United Nations Educational, Scientific and Cultural Organization. Available at http://unesdoc.unesco.org/images/0013/001362/136246e.pdf, accessed on 19 August 2016.

Van der Merwe, A. (2009) "A Theoretical Framework for the Characterization of Pathological Speech Sensorimotor Control." In M.R. McNeil (ed.) *Clinical Management of Sensorimotor Speech Disorders, 2nd Edition*. New York, NY: Thieme.

van Kleeck, A. (1994) "Potential cultural bias in training parents as conversational partners with their children who have delays in language development." *American Journal of Speech-Language Pathology 3*, 67–78.

van Kleeck, A. and Schuele, C. (1987) "Precursors to literacy: Normal development." *Topics in Language Disorders 7*, 2, 13–31.

Vukelich, C., Christie, J., and Enz, B. (2002) *Helping Young Children Learn Language and Literacy*. Boston, MA: Allyn and Bacon.

Weiss, A.L. (2014) "Comprehension of Language." In N. Capone Singleton and B.B. Shulman (eds) *Language Development: Foundations, Processes, and Clinical Applications, 2nd Edition*. Burlington, MA: Jones and Bartlett Learning.

Wenig, M. (2003) *YogaKids: Educating the Whole Child Through Yoga*. New York, NY: Stewart, Tabori & Chang.

Westby, C. (2000) "A Scale for Assessing Development of Children's Play." In K. Gitlin-Weiner, A. Sandgrund, and C. Schaefer (eds) *Play Diagnosis and Assessment, 2nd Edition*. New York, NY: John Wiley & Sons, Inc.

White, L.S. (2012) "Reducing stress in school-age girls through mindful yoga." *Journal of Pediatric Health Care 26*, 1, 45–56.

Whitehurst, G.J. and Lonigan, C.J. (1998) "Child development and emergent literacy." *Child Development 69*, 3, 848–872.

Willcutt, E.G. and Pennington, B.F. (2000) "Comorbidity of reading disability and attention deficit/hyperactivity disorder: Differences by gender and subtype." *Journal of Learning Disabilities 33*, 2, 179–191.

Williams, N. (2010) *Yoga Therapy for Every Special Child.* London: Jessica Kingsley Publishers.

Willis, J. (2006) *Research-Based Strategies to Ignite Student Learning: Insights from a Neurologist and Classroom Teacher.* Alexandria, VA: Association for Supervision and Curriculum Development.

Wills, R. (2015) "The interthoracic connection." *Respiratory Therapy 10*, 2, 24–26.

Wills, R., Seberg, S., and Economides, S. (2014) *The Inter-Thoracic Connection: SLP Collaboration with PT and RT for Improving Breathing Mechanics.* Lincoln, NE: Madonna Rehabilitation Hospital. Available at www.passy-muir.com/sites/default/files/pdf/asha_2015_madonna_presentation.pdf, accessed on 9 August 2016.

Yaffa, G. and Yaffa, A. (n.d.) *Teaching Rainbow Kids Yoga.* Australia: Rainbow Kids Yoga.

Yoga Journal and *Yoga Alliance* (2016) *Yoga in America Study. Yoga Journal* and *Yoga Alliance.* Available at http://media.yogajournal.com/wp-content/uploads/2016-Yoga-in-America-Study-Comprehensive-RESULTS.pdf, accessed on 16 August 2016.

Yurtkuran, M., Alp, A., Yurtkuran, M., and Dilek, K. (2007) "A modified yoga-based exercise program in hemodialysis patients: A randomized controlled study." *Complementary Therapies in Medicine 15*, 3, 164–171.

Index

Page numbers in *italics* refer to figures and tables.

CPI Antony Rowe
Eastbourne, UK
June 20, 2023